Essentials of Assessing Infants, Toddlers, and Preschoolers

Essentials

of Assessing Infants, Toddlers, and Preschoolers

Brittany A. Dale, Joseph R. Engler,
and Vincent C. Alfonso

WILEY

Published by John Wiley & Sons, Inc., Hoboken, New Jersey.
Published simultaneously in Canada.

Library of Congress Cataloging-in-Publication Data Applied for:

Paperback ISBN: 9781394152070

Cover Design: Wiley
Cover Image: © Robert/Adobe Stock

Set in 11.5/14pt AGaramondPro by Straive, Pondicherry, India

To my Alan, my forever teammate, partner, and love, thank you for always
believing in me even when I may not believe in myself. You always
encourage me to pursue my dreams and to stay persistent as I work
toward them. To Isaac, you have been the greatest gift, and I am honored
to be your mom. Your energy, laughter, and kindness brighten my world.
You both are my heart, my strength, and my inspiration.

-Brittany

Although titles have never been important to me, there is one that I cherish
and has fundamentally changed my life. The title is 'dad.' To Elin and
Siena, thank you for giving me this title and all the happiness that comes
with it! Every day I pinch myself knowing that I get to share my life with
you. Watching the two of you develop into such wonderful human beings
has truly been a gift. To Calissa, my partner and best friend, thank you for
your steadfast love and support. Every day you model and teach our
children the importance of love, laughter, generosity, forgiveness,
and so much more. I am forever grateful that you chose me.

-Joe

As I near the end of my formal, professional career, there are many
individuals in my life who have guided, mentored, challenged, and cared for
me. The number is high, but the following individuals have been my
closest and longest professional guardian angels and for them I am forever
grateful and dedicate this volume: Anita Batisti, Anthony Cancelli,
Jim Hennessy, Steve Hess, Patricia Killen, Pat Lee, Beth Martin,
Skip Meyers, Bob Niehoff, and Jim Voiss.

-Vinny

CONTENTS

In the paraphrased words of Alexander Pope, "As the twig is bent, so grows the tree." This timeless adage, from his 1732 work *Epistles to Several Persons*, underscores the profound impact of early experiences on a child's development. It is this foundational wisdom that drives the emphasis on infant and early childhood assessment and intervention among psychologists and educators and provides the basis for this book authored by Dale, Engler, and Alfonso. More than a century of developmental research has demonstrated that the experiences of early childhood can shape an individual's future in significant ways. Positive early influences foster robust and healthy development, while adverse conditions can lead to lifelong challenges. This book delves into the critical role of early childhood assessment, identification, education, and intervention toward nurturing healthy children, adolescents, and adults. As the former slave and abolitionist Frederick Douglass aptly stated, "It is easier to build strong children than to repair broken men."

Chapters 2 and 3 of this book highlight the necessity of a combined standardized and clinical approach to validly assess young children. Creating a supportive and engaging environment during assessments is essential to make children feel comfortable and cooperative, as emphasized by Bracken and Theodore (2020a, 2020b). This artful combined clinical and standardized approach to assessment incorporates a variety of crucial factors, including children's temperament styles, cultural contexts, health, and socialization experiences. Given that young children express themselves uniquely and sometimes idiosyncratically, assessments must be flexible and adaptable while maintaining standardized administration to ensure integrity. To enhance the validity and reliability of assessment data, it is crucial to triangulate information through meaningful *in vivo* observations, interviews with teachers and caregivers, and the administration of developmentally appropriate direct assessment tools. Current instrumentation, processes, and procedures are covered herein in a conversant and descriptive manner, making the reader aware of considerable general information while providing salient references for those who seek additional detail.

Chapters 4 and 5 reflect decades of developmental research, which mapped "normal" child development, identified important developmental domains, led to the formation of relevant professional organizations, and revealed myriad common developmental disorders. Arnold Gesell's pioneering work in the assessment and documentation of infant and toddler development was crucial in elucidating the rate and sequence of early childhood developmental milestones. Understanding when these momentous events typically occur helps professionals identify potential issues of concern and determine when interventions might be necessary. Because early childhood years are a critical period of rapid physical, cognitive, linguistic, and social-emotional growth, identifying delays in any area of development—be it language, motor skills, cognition, social-emotional, or adaptive behavior—early in a child's life can lead to timely, evidence-based interventions, ensuring children receive the support they need to thrive.

Assessing young children with low-incidence developmental and medical disorders requires specialized expertise and tools. The Individuals with Disabilities Education Act (IDEA) Part B identifies core developmental areas—cognition, motor skills, language, social-emotional development, and adaptive behavior—that are vital for healthy development. These domains are extensively covered in the literature of professional organizations such as the National Association for the Education of Young Children (NAEYC), the National Association of School Psychologists (NASP), and the American Psychological Association (APA). IDEA Part B legislation aspires to ensure that children with disabilities receive early intervention across these essential domains. To facilitate evidence-based interventions based on developmentally sound assessments, the authors appropriately stress the importance of collaboration among healthcare professionals, educators, and caregivers to provide comprehensive care and support.

Chapter 6 outlines a proactive assessment-intervention approach that may help caregivers and professionals foster children's potential, reduce future learning difficulties, and contribute to better long-term outcomes in education, health, and social skill development. Early identification of developmental issues also supports families by providing caregivers with essential information, identifying community resources, and promoting collaborative strategies to effectively nurture their child's development.

This book, through its seven highly relevant chapters, explores the history and future trends in infant and early childhood assessment and intervention. It also considers the legal requirements and professional guidelines for working with culturally, ethnically, and physically diverse populations of exceptional children. Critically, this book highlights the importance of developmentally appropriate early childhood assessments and evidence-based interventions, emphasizing the essential connection between the two. By delving into these themes, the authors provide a comprehensive understanding of how timely assessments and interventions can shape healthier, more successful futures for children. This book serves as a valuable resource for professionals and caregivers dedicated to supporting the developmental needs of young children.

Bruce A. Bracken, PhD
October 28, 2024, Williamsburg, VA

REFERENCES

Bracken, B. A., & Theodore, L. A. (2020a). Observations of preschool children's assessment-related behaviors. In V. C. Alfonso, B. A. Bracken, & R. J. Nagle (Eds.), *Psychoeducational assessment of preschool children* (5th ed., pp. 33–54). Rutledge.

Bracken, B. A., & Theodore, L. A. (2020b). Creating the optimal preschool testing situation. In V. C. Alfonso, B. A. Bracken, & R. J. Nagle (Eds.), *Psychoeducational assessment of preschool children* (5th ed., pp. 55–76). Rutledge.

"As the twig is bent, so is the tree inclined." The Oxford Dictionary of Phrase and Fable. Retrieved October 15, 2024, from Encyclopedia.com: https://www.encyclopedia.com/humanities/dictionaries-thesauruses-pictures-and-press-releases/twig-bent-so-tree-inclined. Oxford University Press.

One

OVERVIEW OF INFANT, TODDLER, AND PRESCHOOL ASSESSMENT[1]

An ounce of prevention is worth a pound of cure.

Benjamin Franklin

It is important to have a context from which to understand the focus of this volume, which is infant, toddler, and preschool assessment. As such, we begin this volume with the rationale for and importance of early childhood assessment followed by a brief history of infant, toddler, and preschool assessment using several sources of information, including Alfonso et al. (2022), Alfonso, Bracken, et al. (2020), Alfonso, Engler, et al. (2020, 2024), Alfonso, Ruby, et al. (2020), Black and Matula (2000), Goodman (1990), Kelley and Surbeck (2007), and Nagle et al. (2020). Additionally, Sattler (2018) has a very useful summary of the historical milestones in intellectual and developmental assessment.

The interested reader is encouraged to review these sources as well as others, including Chapters 3 and 6 in this volume, to gain a thorough understanding of the history of infant, toddler, and preschool assessment. We begin the chapter by providing a rationale for the importance of early childhood assessment and intervention. Then we provide information on relevant law and advocacy for the assessment of young children. At the end of the chapter, we provide a brief annotated bibliography and a list of early childhood

---

[1] Portions of this chapter were adapted or reproduced with permission from Alfonso et al. (2022). *Essentials of Bayley-4 assessment.* John Wiley & Sons.

Essentials of Assessing Infants, Toddlers, and Preschoolers, First Edition.
Brittany A. Dale, Joseph R. Engler, and Vincent C. Alfonso.
© 2025 John Wiley & Sons, Inc. Published 2025 by John Wiley & Sons, Inc.

resources for further learning. Finally, the Appendix summarizes infant, toddler, and preschool measures by domain and age as a resource for practitioners working with young children. Throughout this volume, we use various terms relevant to the assessment of young children. See Rapid Reference 1.1 for a definition of the most relevant terms.

≡ Rapid Reference 1.1 Key Definitions

Assessment	The process of gathering data to inform decision-making
Evaluation	The interpretation of assessment data to inform decision-making
Measure/Test	A specific assessment tool used for an evaluation of a young child

RATIONALE FOR AND IMPORTANCE OF EARLY CHILDHOOD ASSESSMENT AND INTERVENTION

In this section, we discuss the rationale for and importance of early childhood assessment, highlighting the following: (1) nurturing the youngest of the species, (2) incidence and prevalence of early childhood disorders, (3) effectiveness of early childhood education and intervention, and (4) the use of technology in the delivery of early childhood health services. Although space limitations preclude a lengthy discussion of these topics, our goal is to provide enough scientifically based knowledge so the reader understands the need for and benefits of early childhood assessment and intervention.

Nurturing the Youngest of the Species

Most, if not all animals, in the animal kingdom protect and nurture the youngest of their species, at least until they can care for themselves. Popular television shows such as *Earth Odyssey* (2019-present), *Wild Child* (2021-present), Jack Hanna's *Into the Wild* (2007-2020), and many others fascinate children and adults alike as they learn about survival in the wild and how young animals are raised by their adult parents. In 2005, the movie *March of the Penguins* was released to critical acclaim, and we learned how adult male and female emperor penguins share the responsibility of raising their young.

Despite some evidence to the contrary, such as mass shootings of children in the United States and war-torn countries where children are inexplicable casualties, adult male and female human beings (i.e., *homo sapiens*) nurture their children with great care and love at least until age 18 years when they become legal adults. Indeed, *homo sapiens* are members of the animal kingdom and as such, share many of the characteristics of other animals. For example, the famous zoologist Desmond Morris wrote extensively in *The Naked Ape* (1967) on how *homo sapiens* are like other great apes (i.e., primates) in their care for the young. Most of us are also familiar with another ethologist, Jane Goodall, who studied chimpanzees' social and family interactions for more than six decades.

The work of several psychologists such as John Bowlby (e.g., 1988), Mary Ainsworth et al. (e.g., 1978), and Harry Harlow (e.g., 1958), to name a few, influenced our thinking of attachment, the parent–child bond, and the importance of healthy early child development for success later in life. Although some researchers and scholars question the influence of or need for parents in children's lives (e.g., Harris, 2000), most believe that parents (or at least loving, nurturing adults) are important influences in a young child's life (see, e.g., Bronfenbrenner, 1977, 1986; Bronfenbrenner & Morris, 2006; Collins et al., 2000; Davis-Kean et al., 2021; National Academies of Sciences, Engineering, and Medicine, 2016; Wilder, 2014).

In addition to parents or primary caregivers, there are many other influences on young children's development sometimes referred to as spheres of influence. Some of these spheres include friendships (e.g., Harris, 2000), extended family members such as grandparents (e.g., Mayer, 2002), immediate physical context (e.g., Evans, 2021), environmental factors such as national and world climate change and toxins (e.g., Koger et al., 2005; Vergunst & Berry, 2022), and socioeconomics including financial and other resources (e.g., Aber et al., 1997; Aboud & Yousafzai, 2015; Brooks-Gunn & Duncan, 1997; Chen, 2012; Evans, 2004; Evans & Cassells, 2014; Evans & Kim, 2013; Evans et al., 2013; Fernald et al., 2009; Frankenhuis & Nettle, 2020; Maholmes & King, 2012; McLoyd, 1998; The World Bank, 2015). Later in this chapter, we address the importance of early childhood assessment and intervention as they relate to some of the influences stated here.

Before we turn to the incidence and prevalence of early childhood disorders, it is worth noting the mounting evidence contrary to John Locke's concept of the young child as a *blank slate* (1690/1947). Today we know and every year we learn more about the capabilities of infants, toddlers, and preschoolers (see, e.g., Feldman, 2019 and Pinker, 2002). Once thought of as organisms upon which the world shapes and influences them in a unidirectional manner, we have learned how capable these youngest members of the species are as well as how they shape and influence adults in their lives. For example, de Barbaro and Fausey (2022) described a study that involved infants wearing audio recorders, accelerometers, and cameras to capture their experiences in everyday life. These researchers concluded that "The striking heterogeneity of experiences—the fact that there is no meaningfully 'representative' hour of a day, instance of a category, interaction context, or infant—inspires next steps in theory and practice that embrace the complex, dynamic, and multiple pathways of human development" (p. 28).

> **DON'T FORGET 1.1**
>
> In addition to parents or primary caregivers, there are many other influences on young children's development, sometimes referred to as spheres of influence.

Indeed, human development is complex and dynamic and includes multiple pathways. Recent research in fields of study such as biology, cognitive science, medical physics, neuroanatomy, neuropsychology, obstetrics, and others indicate this clearly (e.g., Adolph, 2019; Aylward, 2020; Cesario et al., 2020; DiPietro, 2000; Glynn & Sandman, 2011; Lee et al., 2018; Perone et al., 2021; Reid & Dunn, 2021; Romeo et al. 2018; UNICEF, 2017). It is incumbent upon early childhood practitioners to engage in professional development activities such as attending conferences, viewing webinars, reading articles in a variety of fields, and consulting with other professionals to remain abreast of the myriad advances we know about young children's capabilities and the influences on early childhood development. We turn now to the incidence and prevalence of early childhood disorders and disability categories.

Incidence and Prevalence of Early Childhood Disorders and Disability Categories

There are dozens, if not hundreds, of early childhood disorders depending on what source or diagnostic/classification system the practitioner uses. The three most common diagnostic/classification systems are the *Individuals with*

Disabilities Education Improvement Act (IDEA, 2004)[2], the *Diagnostic and Statistical Manual of Mental Disorders, Fifth Edition, Text Revision* (DSM-5, TR; American Psychiatric Association [APA], 2022), and *International Classification of Diseases, Tenth Edition* (IDC-10; World Health Organization [WHO], 2016). Practitioners working in early childhood educational settings use IDEA as their classification system or guide when determining eligibility for early intervention or special education services because it is tied to government early intervention funding and other resources and is the model to be used in public education settings. That said, there is almost no one-to-one correspondence between disability categories found in IDEA and disorders found in the DSM-5-TR or ICD-10.

CAUTION 1.1

There is almost no one-to-one correspondence between disability categories found in the IDEA and disorders found in the DSM-5-TR or ICD-10.

As such, we discuss the disability categories found in Parts B and C of IDEA. These disability categories or types are applicable to children ages 3–5 years (Part B) and children ages birth to 2 years (Part C)[3]. Rapid Reference 1.2 includes the 13 disability categories for individuals ages 3–21 years (which, of course, includes children ages 3–5 years). It is important to note that states also have the option of classifying a young child, including those between 3 and 5 years, as a child with a developmental delay rather than using the discreet disability categories found in Rapid Reference 1.2 (Danaher, 2011). Although this modification to IDEA was well-received in the early childhood community, it made the task of counting children under the 13 disability categories very challenging. Moreover, unlike preschool children with disabilities served in Part B of IDEA, children in early intervention (Part C) are not classified by their disability category or type. They are classified as having an established condition or developmental delay (McWilliam, 2016).

---

[2] Throughout this volume, we refer to the *Individuals with Disabilities Education Improvement Act* of 2004 as IDEA since this acronym has persisted in within schools and in the literature.

[3] Chapter 5 addresses other classifying conditions or disorders that could fall under one of the IDEA classification conditions. For example, young children with Down Syndrome have an intellectual disability and would most likely be served under the classification of *intellectual disability* in IDEA.

Boyle et al. (2011) determined the prevalence of developmental disabilities in children in the United States and in selected populations from 1997 to 2008. Although they included individuals between ages 3 and 17, they concluded that the prevalence of any developmental disability increased from 12.84% to 15.04% over the 12-year period. Autism, attention deficit hyperactivity disorder, and other developmental delays increased, whereas hearing loss showed a significant decline. These trends were found in all sociodemographic subgroups, except for autism in non-Hispanic black children.

≋ Rapid Reference 1.2 Thirteen IDEA Disability Categories Applicable for Children Ages 3–5 Years

- Deaf Blindness
- Traumatic Brain Injury
- Visual Impairment
- Emotional Disturbance
- Orthopedic Impairment
- Multiple Disabilities
- Hearing Impairment
- Specific Learning Disability
- Intellectual Disability
- Other Health Impairment
- Autism
- Developmental Delay
- Speech or Language Impairment

The United States Department of Education (USDOE) provided data on the number of 3–5-year-old children with disabilities served under IDEA, Part B, from 2010 to 2018 (USDOE, 2020b). For example, in 2010, nearly 179,000 3-year-olds were served, while in the same year, nearly 263,000 and 297,000 4 and 5-year-olds, respectively, were served. Seven years later in 2018, the respective numbers were 192,000, 283,000, and 339,000. As can be seen in these numbers, more children at each age were served in 2018 than in 2010. In 2018–2019, 6.75% of 3–5-year-olds in the United States were served under Part B of IDEA. An additional percentage of interest in 2018–2019 is that 8.43% of students with disabilities, aged 3 through 5, were English Learners. Rapid Reference 1.3 includes the 13 disability categories for individuals ages 3–5 years along with the corresponding number of children served in each category for the year 2018–2019.

≡ Rapid Reference 1.3 Thirteen IDEA Disability Categories Applicable to Children Ages 3–5 Years and Number of Children Served in Each Category in 2018–2019

- Deaf Blindness – 181
- Traumatic Brain Injury – 1,158
- Visual Impairment – 2,697
- Emotional Disturbance – 2,882
- Orthopedic Impairment – 5,111
- Multiple Disabilities – 7,702
- Hearing Impairment – 8,865
- Specific Learning Disability – 8,909
- Intellectual Disability – 13,369
- Other Health Impairment – 26,104
- Autism – 92,990
- Developmental Delay – 307,335
- Speech or Language Impairment – 337,707

Source: Adapted from U.S. Department of Education, EDFacts Data Warehouse (EDW): "IDEA Part B Child Count and Educational Environments Collection," 2018–2019. http://go.usa.gov/xdp4T.

According to the USDOE Office of Special Education Programs, the number of children receiving services under Part C of IDEA rose from 194,000 in 2010 to more than 400,000 in 2022 (USDOE, 2020a). The amount of money in millions of dollars rose from 117 in 1991 to nearly 500 in 2022. Finally, the amount of dollars per child increased from 603 in 1991 to more than 1200 in 2022 (ECTA, 2024). These data indicate clearly that the USDOE recognizes young children (birth to 2 years) at risk for developmental delay and is allocating much-needed financial resources to support their success. It is important to note, however, that these data reflect the number of children receiving services. Some researchers indicate there are many more children in this age range who are eligible for services, but for many reasons, are not receiving them (e.g., Barger et al., 2018; Rosenberg et al., 2008; Twardzik et al., 2017).

> **CAUTION 1.2**
>
> There are many more young children (birth to 2 years) who are eligible for services, but for many reasons, are not receiving them.

If we believe as a species that we should be caring for our young and that the number of young children (birth to 5 years) eligible for early childhood intervention services is increasing each year due, in part, to the child find element in IDEA, it seems reasonable to ask if early childhood education and intervention are effective. We turn to this topic next but offer here a resounding answer of *yes* as the data in support of the effectiveness of early childhood education and intervention are nearly indisputable.

Effectiveness of Early Childhood Education and Early Intervention

There are few guarantees in life and perhaps even fewer facts or truths in psychology or education. However, in the past several decades research via a myriad of studies has demonstrated the benefits of early childhood education and early intervention (Alfonso, Ruby, et al., 2020; Avellar et al., 2013; Guralnick, 1997; Hebbeler et al., 2007; Hughes & Quinn, 2020; Karoly et al., 2001, 2005; Raines et al., 2020; Ramey & Ramey, 1998, 2004; Ramey et al., 2014; Redden et al., 1999, 2001; Schweinhart & Weikart, 1998; Trohanis, 2008; Zigler & Muenchow, 1992). For example, there is substantial agreement that high-quality early intervention programs for vulnerable infants and toddlers can reduce the incidence of future problems in their learning, behavior, and health status and that intervention is likely to be more effective and less costly when it is provided earlier in life rather than later (Center on the Developing Child at Harvard University, 2008, 2010; National Early Childhood Technical Assistance Center, 2011). Moreover, these facts or truths seem to resonate with individuals from all walks of life, political parties, and professions who engage in working with young children (e.g., Division for Early Childhood [DEC] of the Council for Exceptional Children, 2014; National Association for the Education of Young Children [NAEYC], 2020; National Association of School Psychologists, 2015; Public Laws 99–457, 101–476, 105-17, and 108–446).

Bann et al. (2016) demonstrated that early intervention altered trajectories of cognitive development among children from disadvantaged backgrounds. That is, children from low-resource families receiving a home-based intervention focused on motor, social, and language development, had 36-month cognitive development scores statistically indistinguishable from those of children from high-resource families. Litt et al. (2018) found that early intervention services improved school-age functional outcomes among neonatal intensive care unit graduates, and Noyes-Grosser et al. (2018) demonstrated that children with autism spectrum disorder showed reduced maladaptive behaviors and improved social and communication skills and some also made progress on IDEA Part C child outcome indicators. In addition, families of children with autism spectrum disorder reported that early intervention helped them achieve many outcomes identified as important to them.

Two early childhood programs or projects deserve special mention here: The High/Scope Perry Preschool Project (Schweinhart et al., 2005; Weikart, 1967, 1970) and The Carolina Abecedarian Project/Approach (Ramey & Campbell, 1984; Ramey & Ramey, 1999; Ramey et al., 1976, 1981, 1985, 2012, 2014). The High/Scope Perry Preschool Project was a scientific experiment in Ypsilanti, Michigan, for young children to help them avoid school failure and many other challenges. It identified the short- and long-term effects of a high-quality preschool education program for young children living in poverty from 1962 through 1967. One hundred twenty-three African American children were determined to be at high risk for school failure as indicated by socioeconomic and standardized assessment measures. Fifty-eight were assigned to a program group that received a high-quality preschool program at ages 3 and 4 years, and 65 of them were assigned to another group that received no preschool program. All children were randomly assigned and as such, most scholars and researchers believe it was the children's preschool experience that explained the group differences in education, income, crime, family relationships, and health. That is, the experimental group (those children who received the preschool program) outperformed the control group (those children who did not receive the preschool program) on each of these variables. The children (now adults) have been followed for decades with a missing data rate of only 6% across all measures.

The Carolina Abecedarian Project was like the High/Scope Perry Preschool Project in that its aim was to alter the life trajectory of young children from low-resource environments by providing them with high-quality early education. One hundred eleven infants from low-resource families participated with 57 receiving high-quality early childhood education and 54 receiving supports (e.g., social services, health care), but no high-quality education. Specifically, in the Carolina Abecedarian Project.

"Control groups of children who did not receive the Abecedarian Approach received the same levels of support as the educationally treated children for additional health care, free and unlimited nutritional supports, and active social work services to the families, as well as timely referrals when any problems were detected or suspected. Because the control groups received these multiple supports, the research findings provided a strong basis for concluding that it was the educational features of the Abecedarian Approach that produced the documented differences between the children in the experimental groups and the comparison groups . . ." (Ramey et al., 2014, p. 441).

As with the High/Scope Perry Preschool Project, there have been several follow-up studies with the original Carolina Abecedarian Project participants into adulthood. Once again, those children (now adults) who received the high-quality early childhood educational experience demonstrated significant differences (i.e., higher or better) in cognitive functioning, academic skills, educational attainment, employment, parenthood, and social adjustment (Campbell & Ramey, 1994; Campbell et al., 2001, 2002). According to Ramey et al. (2014),

"The issue of efficacy of early childhood education for high-risk children is settled. Yes, we can prevent a great deal of developmental delay. For us, the most pressing questions in early childhood education now become: (1) comparative efficacy of different early childhood programs, (2) differential response to treatment, (3) scale-up of effective programs, and (4) standards for programs aimed at preventing developmental delay. It feels good to move beyond the efficacy issue that dominated thinking about early childhood education for half a century" (p. 468).

> **DON'T FORGET 1.2**
>
> The data in support of the effectiveness of early childhood education and intervention are nearly indisputable.

The importance of early childhood education and early intervention as explicated above, together with major advances in prenatal care, pediatric medicine, neuropsychology, and neuroimaging, have highlighted the need for reliable and valid assessment of infants, toddlers, and preschoolers (e.g., Aylward, 2010, 2020; Brito, Fifer et al., 2019; Kelley & Surbeck, 2007; McCloskey et al., 2020; Snow & Van Hemel, 2008). Many scholars, researchers, practitioners, and organizations believe there are several purposes of infant, toddler, and preschool assessment. For example, Nagle et al. (2020) integrated other sources such as NAEYC, DEC, and individual scholarly works to summarize the major purposes, which they state are the following: (1) screening, (2) diagnosis and eligibility determination, (3) individual program planning and monitoring, and (4) program evaluation.

Typical domains of development requiring assessment include cognitive abilities and processes, motor skills, speech and language skills, social–emotional behavior, and adaptive behavior (Alfonso, Bracken, et al., 2020; Alfonso, Engler, et al., 2020; Bellman et al., 2013; Brassard & Boehm, 2007; NAEYC, 2020; Snow & Van Hemel 2008). Additional assessment domains include intrauterine (prenatal and perinatal), physical, parenting, parenting stress, and play. Play is particularly important to assess as there is ample evidence regarding the benefits of play on the young child's developing brain, social interactions, and cognitive functioning (e.g., Kelly-Vance & Ryalls, 2020).

Many domains of functioning are assessed with developmental measures such as the Bayley Scales of Infant and Toddler Development, Fourth Edition (Bayley–4; Bayley & Aylward, 2019). For example, Alfonso et al. (2022) state that the Bayley–4 may be used for the following purposes: (1) to identify children with developmental delay, (2) research related to individual program planning and monitoring and program evaluation, and (3) to monitor a child's developmental progress. The Appendix provides a summary of infant, toddler, and preschool measures by domain and age as a resource for practitioners working with young children. The last topic in this section is the burgeoning use of technology in the delivery of early childhood health services.

DON'T FORGET 1.3

Typical domains of development requiring assessment include cognitive abilities and processes, motor skills, speech and language skills, social–emotional behavior, and adaptive behavior.

Use of Technology in the Delivery of Early Childhood Health Services

Given the need to provide early childhood assessment and intervention services to young children as soon as possible, especially for those living in rural areas, the use of technology is becoming an efficient and effective means of delivering these services. For example, Meadan and Daczewitz (2015) described internet-based intervention training for parents of young children with disabilities as a promising service-delivery model. Indeed, although the COVID-19 pandemic had a profound effect on the use of technology in the delivery of early childhood services, including assessment and intervention, teleassessment, telepractice, and telehealth were occurring at least a decade prior or even earlier. For example, Behl et al. (2010) wrote about tele-intervention as the wave of the future that was already in use with children and families where a child had hearing loss. In addition, these authors stated, "Many agencies within the United States are using telehealth practices to conduct hearing evaluations on infants who do not pass their newborn hearing screening test" (p. 28). Several years later, Behl et al. (2017) demonstrated the effectiveness of telepractice as a method of delivering early intervention services to families of infants and toddlers who are deaf or hard of hearing. Baharav and Reiser (2010) discussed the use of telepractice in parent training in early autism. They noted several benefits, including treatment effectiveness, adaptability to technology, and client satisfaction with the service.

Still prior to COVID-19, the state of Colorado began allowing the use of telehealth as an option for providers to conduct sessions with children and their caregivers in their Part C early intervention programming (Cole et al., 2019). Sutherland et al. (2018) reported a summary of studies of 284 individuals, ages 19 months to adult, with autism spectrum disorder who received a variety of telehealth services. Their results suggested "that services delivered via telehealth were equivalent to services delivered face to face, and superior to comparison groups without telehealth sessions" (p. 324). There have been studies and reports on the delivery of telehealth services for individuals across the lifespan, including young children, that took place during COVID-19. For example, Andrews et al. (2020) conducted an integrative review of 18 studies that examined health care providers' and patient satisfaction with telehealth services during COVID-19. They found high levels of satisfaction for patients and health care providers, and many were willing to continue telehealth after the pandemic. In Ore's (2021) review on the effectiveness of telehealth for children with autism spectrum disorder during COVID-19, he concluded, "Evidence from the review indicates that telehealth can be an alternative to face-to-face cognitive assessment. Telehealth may present a feasible and reliable approach to the assessment of language for children with autism spectrum disorders in some circumstances as a primary or adjunct service model" (p. 3).

The interested practitioner may find additional publications worth reading as this section simply touched upon the evidence indicating that telehealth is an effective delivery model for early childhood services. For example, the American Academy of Pediatrics (2020) discusses what is pediatric telehealth, Frye et al. (2022) discusses the implementation of telehealth during COVID-19 as well as implications for providing behavioral health services to pediatric patients, and Atiles et al. (2021) reports on challenges faced by international early childhood professionals during COVID-19. Chapter 7 of this volume expands the discussion of the use of technology in the delivery of early childhood services. Now we turn to a brief history of infant, toddler, and preschool assessment.

BRIEF HISTORY OF INFANT, TODDLER, AND PRESCHOOL ASSESSMENT

Although it may seem that early childhood assessment has been a common practice for centuries, it is only about 200 years old (Kelley & Surbeck, 2007). Influences on early childhood assessment include dozens of individuals, but a few are worth mentioning by name. For example, the precursor to early childhood assessment and developmental psychology may be attributed to the naturalistic observations of Johann Heinrich Pestalozzi in the 18th century and G. Stanley Hall, who is regarded as the father of developmental psychology and was the first president of the American Psychological Association (APA; Black & Matula, 2000). In the latter part of the 19th century, Sir Francis Galton, a cousin to Charles Darwin, constructed "tests of memory, motor, and sensory functions to differentiate between high and low achievers" (Kelley & Surbeck, 2007, p. 4). As a result, Galton became known as the father of mental testing.

Perhaps the most famous early contributor to the practice of early childhood assessment, especially the assessment of mental ability or intelligence, was Alfred Binet, who with Theodore Simon, created the Binet-Simon Scale for measuring the intelligence of school children (Binet & Simon, 1905). It was translated to English from French by Henry Goddard (a student of G. Stanley Hall), who also believed in the importance of early diagnosis, systematic testing, and special placements for school-aged students who evidenced learning difficulties (Kelley & Surbeck, 2007). The Binet-Simon Scale became the template for most, if not all, intelligence, and cognitive batteries to the present day.

The child study movement of the early 1900s, which saw a proliferation of funding, studies, and assessments of school-aged children focusing on intelligence, memory, perception, emotion, personality, and motivation, influenced early childhood psychologists to begin paying attention to infants, toddlers, and preschoolers (Black & Matula, 2000; Kelley & Surbeck, 2007). Among the most famous and influential early childhood (infant) psychologists was Arnold Gesell, who was also a pediatrician by training. Some refer to him as the grandfather of infant assessment (Goodman, 1990). According to Black and Matula (2000), Gesell, who was greatly influenced by Charles Darwin, "compiled a schedule of tasks for infants 4, 6, 9, 12, and 18 months of age and 2, 3, 4, and 5 years of age" (Gesell, 1925, p. 3). These Developmental Schedules continued to be used for decades in various circles, especially by medical personnel (Goodman, 1990), and influenced the first infant intelligence tests such as the Cattell Infant Intelligence Scale (Cattell, 1940), Griffiths Mental Development Scale for Testing Babies from Birth to Two Years (Griffiths, 1951), and Bayley Scales of Infant Development (Bayley, 1969). Black and Matula (2000) state, "These early assessments were designed to catalog an infant's level of development at various ages and to establish normative data" (p. 4). Unfortunately, they did not predict future functioning as many thought they would, which called into question their utility (Goodman, 1990).

In the past 50 years, several factors or variables have influenced the importance of early childhood assessment as well as the proliferation of measures or instruments to accomplish the task of reliable and valid assessment. Perhaps the most salient are the following cited by Black and Matula (2000): (1) many premature and medically vulnerable infants are surviving, which typically necessitates assessment, (2) infant assessments are needed to determine if infants are developing at an expected rate or evidencing a developmental delay, (3) whether young children meet the criteria for early intervention services, and (4) whether early intervention is effective in improving their rate of development. Additional factors that continue to influence the importance of early childhood assessment are law and advocacy that are discussed next.

> **DON'T FORGET 1.4**
>
> In the past 50 years, several factors or variables have influenced the importance of early childhood assessment as well as the proliferation of measures or instruments to accomplish the task of reliable and valid assessment.

LAW AND ADVOCACY

Earlier in this chapter, we discussed the effectiveness of early childhood education and intervention as an important rationale for early childhood assessment and corresponding intervention. Concomitant with the body of evidence in support of early childhood education and assessment is the increasingly greater focus of legislation and policy on assessing young children (Alfonso et al., 2024). Typically, practitioners assess young children suspected of having a developmental delay or a specific disorder (e.g., autism and intellectual disability). However, there is ample enthusiasm around universal pre-k, full-day kindergarten, and early childhood screening as means of prevention and promotion of success in the early grades.

Early Childhood Assessment and Intervention Public Laws

In 1986, Congress passed the 1986 amendment (PL 99–457) to the Education for all Handicapped Children Act (PL 94–142, 1975). This law extended downward the rights and provisions of school-aged children with disabilities to children from 3 to 5 years of age, as well as infants and toddlers who were at risk for developmental delay. When Congress reauthorized PL 94–142 in 1990, it renamed it the Individuals with Disabilities Education Act (IDEA) known as PL 108–446. It was again reauthorized in 2004 as the Individuals with Disabilities Education Improvement Act, but it continues to be known as IDEA. As stated earlier in this chapter Part B, Section 619 of IDEA includes amendments such as ensuring free and appropriate special education services for preschoolers aged 3–5 years and allows individual states to use a broad definition of disability for children 3–9 years of age using the term "developmental delay" to identify a child who is experiencing delays in one or more areas of development. Areas of delay include physical, cognitive, communication, social or emotional, and/or adaptive behavior domains.

Part C of IDEA included incentives for states to develop and provide comprehensive early intervention services for infants and toddlers with disabilities and their families. These young children demonstrate developmental delays or have diagnosed conditions with a high probability of resulting in developmental delay (Alfonso et al., 2024). The IDEA also included more language and emphasis on transitional services from Part C to Part B and a focus on scientifically based academic and behavioral interventions, including early literacy interventions (Alfonso et al., 2024; McBride et al., 2011; McWilliam, 2016). Part C also mandated a multidisciplinary assessment of the infant or toddler's strengths and weaknesses as well as family-directed assessment, "or an understanding of the resources, priorities, and concerns of the family as well as the identification of the supports and services necessary in order to help the family meet the developmental needs of the infant and toddler" (Alfonso et al., 2024).

Early childhood practitioners also engage in assessment to ensure academic success, even when there is no suspected developmental delay or diagnosable condition. For example, in 2015, the No Child Left Behind Act (NCLB; PL 107–110) was replaced by the Every Student Succeeds Act (ESSA) or PL 114-95. The purpose of the ESSA was to expand access to high-quality early learning so that every child begins kindergarten ready to learn and "to provide all children significant opportunity to receive a fair, equitable, and high-quality education, and to close educational achievement gaps" (Sec. 1001) (Alfonso et al., 2024). ESSA includes funds dedicated to improving the coordination, quality, and access to early childhood education. As such, school or academic readiness once again became familiar terms in the education law, and advocacy literatures. Concomitantly, there has been an increase in publicly funded preschool programs and assessment has been used to demonstrate accountability for various programs (Alfonso et al., 2024; Alfonso, Ruby, et al., 2020).

Head Start and Early Head Start

We would be remiss if we did not write about two of the most important and successful early childhood programs of the past nearly 60 and 30 years, respectfully. These programs are Head Start (which, in some ways, is the precursor to the federal legislation described above) and Early Head Start. In short, these programs were/are designed to provide high-quality early childhood education and care that have a positive impact on young children's, especially those from low-income households, cognitive, language, and social development (Raines et al., 2020).

The roots of Head Start[4] date back to 1965 when President Lyndon B. Johnson declared the war on poverty. Drs. Robert Cooke and Edward Zigler were instrumental in launching Head Start, which established performance standards in 1975 and began offering full-day and full-year services in 1998. In 2007, the Improving Head Start for School Readiness Act was reauthorized. Several provisions were included in this act to ensure the delivery of high-quality early childhood education and care. In the years that followed, additional changes were made to Head Start and Early Head Start, including the Designation Renewal System and revised Program Performance Standards. The Head Start Program serves more than 1 million children and families each year and since 1965 has served more than 36 million children and families. It is administered by the Administration for Children and Families in the Department of Health and Human Services. An excellent review of the history of many early childhood laws is provided by Raines et al. (2020). McBride et al. (2011) cover special education laws including those that address infants, toddlers, and preschoolers.

SUMMARY

Although early childhood assessment is a relatively new activity for practitioners, it is essential for several reasons as explicated in this chapter. These reasons include nurturing the youngest of the species, the ever-increasing incidence and prevalence of early childhood disorders, the effectiveness of early childhood education and intervention, and the burgeoning use of technology in the delivery of early childhood health services. Early intervention for young children has shown to be a critical tool to ensure that young children at risk for developmental disabilities, medical disorders, and poverty live healthy and productive lives. Despite ideological, economic, political, and other challenges, the USDOE continues to increase funding for early childhood education and intervention. The remaining chapters in this volume provide in-depth

---

[4] Retrieved from: https://www.acf.hhs.gov/ohs/about/history-head-start and https://eclkc.ohs.acf.hhs.gov/about-us/article/head-start-timeline

information on the unique considerations when assessing young children, responsible assessment of young children, the developmental domains to assess and why, low-frequency disorders in young children, linking assessment to intervention, and the future of early childhood assessment.

TEST YOURSELF

1. **When considering early childhood development, which of the following factors does evidence suggest is influential?**
   (a) Caregivers or parents
   (b) Extended family
   (c) Physical context
   (d) All of the above

2. **Since 2010, the incidence of early childhood disorders has:**
   (a) Remained stable
   (b) Decreased
   (c) Increased
   (d) Not been measured

3. **Based on data from 2018–2019, which IDEA disability category includes the highest number of children served?**
   (a) Deaf Blindness
   (b) Speech or Language Impairment
   (c) Developmental Delay
   (d) Intellectual Disability

4. **Evidence for early childhood education and intervention indicates the following:**
   (a) It does not promote positive outcomes
   (b) It is more costly than waiting to intervene in adulthood
   (c) It produces negligible outcomes compared to control groups in most studies
   (d) It promotes an array of positive outcomes across developmental domains

5. **Domains typically assessed in early childhood include:**
   (a) Cognitive functioning
   (b) Social–emotional functioning
   (c) Speech and language skills
   (d) All of the above

6. **Potential benefits of telehealth or teleassessment include:**
   (a) Increased access to rural communities
   (b) More efficient and accessible service delivery
   (c) A and B
   (d) None of the above

7. **The following statements are true regarding technology in the delivery of early childhood services except:**
   (a) Should fully supplant the use of in-person early childhood services
   (b) Has been utilized for more than two decades
   (c) Can be an effective service delivery model for clients with autism spectrum disorder
   (d) May be integrated within early intervention programming

8. **Who is regarded as the father of developmental psychology?**
   (a) Alfred Binet
   (b) G. Stanley Hall
   (c) Nancy Bayley
   (d) Arnold Gesell

9. **Which two programs represent the importance and success of early childhood education programs?**
   (a) Head Start
   (b) Early Head Start
   (c) A and B
   (d) None of the above

10. **Which component of IDEA incentivizes states to develop early intervention services for children with disabilities?**
    (a) Part C
    (b) Every Student Succeeds Act (ESSA)
    (c) Part B
    (d) None of the above

Answers: 1. d; 2. c; 3. b; 4. d; 5. d; 6. c; 7. a; 8. b; 9. c; 10. a

REFERENCES

Aber, J. L., Bennett, N. G., Conley, D. C., & Li, J. (1997). The effects of poverty on child health and development. *Annual Review of Public Health, 18*(1), 463–483.

Aboud, F. E., & Yousafzai, A. K. (2015). Global health and development in early childhood. *Annual Review of Psychology, 66*(1), 433–457. https://doi.org/10.1146/annurev-psych-010814-015128

Adolph, K. E. (2019). An ecological approach to learning in (not and) development. *Human Development, 63*(3/4), 180–201. https://doi.org/10.1159/000503823

Ainsworth, M. D., Blehar, M. C., Waters, E., & Wall, S. (1978). *Patterns of attachment: Assess in the strange situation.* Lawrence Erlbaum.

Alfonso, V. C., Bracken, B. A., & Nagle, R. J. (2020). *Psychoeducational assessment of preschool children* (5th ed.). Routledge. https://doi.org/10.4324/9780429054099

Alfonso, V. C., Engler, J. R., & Lepore, J. C. C. (2020). Assessing and evaluating young children: Developmental domains and methods. In V. C. Alfonso & G. J. DuPaul (Eds.), *Healthy development in young children: Evidence-based interventions for early education* (pp. 13–44). American Psychological Association. https://doi.org/10.1037/0000197-002

Alfonso, V. C., Engler, J. R., & Stavrou, E. (2024). Assessment of preschoolers and school readiness. In L. A. Theodore, B. A. Bracken, & M. A. Bray (Eds.), *School psychology desk reference* (pp. 63–79). Oxford University Press.

Alfonso, V. C., Engler, J. R., & Turner, A. D. (2022). *Essentials of Bayley-4 assessment.* John Wiley & Sons.

Alfonso, V. C., Ruby, S., Wissel, A. M., & Davari, J. (2020). School psychologists in early childhood settings. In F. C. Worrell, T. L. Hughes, & D. D. Dixson (Eds.), *The Cambridge handbook of applied school psychology* (pp. 579–597). Cambridge University Press.

American Academy of Pediatrics (AAP). (2020). What is telehealth? Retrieved November 16, 2024 from https://www.aap.org/en-us/professional-resources/practicetransformation/telehealth/Pages/What-is-Telehealth.aspx.

American Psychiatric Association. (2022). *Diagnostic and statistical manual of mental disorders* (5th ed., text rev.). https://doi.org/10.1176/appi.books.9780890425787

Andrews, E., Berghofer, K., Long, J., Prescott, A., & Caboral-Stevens, M. (2020). Satisfaction with the use of telehealth during COVID-19: An integrative review. *International Journal of Nursing Study Advances, 2,* 100008. https://doi.org/10.1016/j.ijnsa.2020.100008

Atiles, A. M., Chavarría, V. A., Dias, M. J. A., & Zúñiga León, I. M. (2021). International responses to COVID-19: Challenges faced by early childhood professionals. *European Early Childhood Education Research Journal, 29*(1), 66–78. https://doi.org/10.1080/1350293X.2021.1872674

Avellar, S., Paulsell, D., SamaMiller, E., & Del Grosso, P. (2013). Home visiting evidence of effectiveness review: Executive summary. Office of Planning, Research and Evaluation, Administration for Children and Families, U.S. Department of Health and Human Services. Retrieved from https://www.acf.hhs.gov/sites/default/files/documents/opre/HomVEE_Executive%20Summary%20August%202017.pdf.

Aylward, G. P. (2010). Methodological considerations in neurodevelopmental outcome studies of infants born prematurely. In I. C. Nosarti, R. Murray, & M. Hack (Eds.), *Neurodevelopmental outcomes of preterm birth from childhood to adult life* (pp. 164–175). Cambridge University Press. https://doi.org/10.1017/CBO9780511712166

Aylward, G. P. (2020). *Bayley 4 clinical use and interpretation.* Academic Press.

Baharav, E., & Reiser, C. (2010). Using tele practice in parent training in early autism. *Telemedicine Journal and E-Health, 16*(6), 727–731. https://doi.org/10.1089/tmj.2010.0029

Bann, C. M., Wallander, J. L., Do, B., Thorsten, V., Pasha, O., Biasini, F. J., Bellad, R., Goudar, S., Chomba, E., McClure, E., & Carlo, W. A. (2016). Home-based early intervention and the influence of family resources on cognitive development. *Pediatrics, 137*(4), e20153766.

Barbaro, K., & Fausey, C. M. (2022). Ten lessons about infants' everyday experiences. *Current Directions in Psychological Science, 31*(1), 28–33.

Barger, R. C., Simmons, C. A., & Wolf, R. (2018). A systematic review of Part C early identification studies. *Topics in Early Childhood Special Education, 38*(1), 4–16. https://doi.org/10.1177/0271121416678664

Bayley, N. (1969). *The Bayley scales of infant development*. Psychological Corporation.

Bayley, N., & Aylward, G. P. (2019). *Bayley scales of infant and toddler development* (4th ed.). Pearson.

Behl, B. K., Cook, G., Barrett, T., Callow-Heusser, C., Brooks, B. M., Dawson, P., Quigley, S., & White, K. R. (2017). A multisite study evaluating the benefits of early intervention via telepractice. *Infants and Young Children, 30*(2), 147–161. https://doi.org/10.1097/IYC.0000000000000090

Behl, D. D., Houston, K. T., Guthrie, W. S., & Guthrie, N. K. (2010). Tele-intervention: The wave of the future fits families' lives today. *The Exceptional Parent, 40*(12).

Bellman, M., Byrne, O., & Sege, R. (2013). Developmental assessment of children. *British Medical Journal, 346*(7891), 31–35. https://doi.org/10.1136/bmj.e8687

Binet, A., & Simon, T. (1905). Méthodes nouvelles pour le diagnostic du niveau intellectuel des anormaux. *L'Année Psychologique, 11*(1), 191–244.

Black, M., & Matula, K. (2000). *Essentials of Bayley scales of infant development-II assessment*. John Wiley & Sons.

Bowlby, J. (1988). *A secure base: Parent-child attachment and healthy human development*. Basic Books.

Boyle, B. S., Schieve, L. A., Cohen, R. A., Blumberg, S. J., Yeargin-Allsopp, M., Visser, S., & Kogan, M. D. (2011). Trends in the prevalence of developmental disabilities in US children, 1997–2008. *Pediatrics, 127*(6), 1034–1042. https://doi.org/10.1542/peds.2010-2989

Brassard, M. R., & Boehm, A. E. (2007). *Preschool assessment: Principles and practices*. Guilford Press.

Brito, N. H., Fifer, W. P., Amso, D., Barr, R., Bell, M. A., Calkins, S., Flynn, A., Montgomery-Downs, H. E., Oakes, L. M., Richards, J. E., Samuelson, L. M., & Colombo, J. (2019). Beyond the Bayley: Neurocognitive assessments of development during infancy and toddlerhood. *Developmental Neuropsychology, 44*(2), 220–247. https://doi.org/10.1080/87565641.2018.1564310

Bronfenbrenner, U. (1977). Toward an experimental ecology of human development. *American Psychologist, 32*(7), 513.

Bronfenbrenner, U. (1986). Ecology of the family as a context for human development: Research perspectives. *Developmental Psychology, 22*(6), 723–742. https://doi.org/10.1037/0012-1649.22.6.723

Bronfenbrenner, U., & Morris, P. A. (2006). The bioecological model of human development. In R. M. Lerner & W. Damon (Eds.), *Handbook of child psychology: Theoretical models of human development* (pp. 793–828). John Wiley & Sons, Inc.

Brooks-Gunn, J., & Duncan, G. J. (1997). The effects of poverty on children. *The Future of Children, 7*(2), 55–71. https://doi.org/10.2307/1602387

Burton, M., Curb, B., Fury, V., Penney, C. & Tear, M., (Executive Producers). (2021 – present). *Wild Child* [TV Series]. National Broadcasting Company.

Campbell, F. A., Pungello, E. P., Miller-Johnson, S., Burchinal, M., & Ramey, C. T. (2001). The development of cognitive and academic abilities: Growth curves from an early childhood educational experiment. *Developmental Psychology, 37*, 231–242.

Campbell, F. A., & Ramey, C. T. (1994). Effects of early intervention on intellectual and academic achievement: A follow-up study of children from low-income families. *Child Development, 65*, 684–698.

Campbell, F. A., Ramey, C. T., Pungello, E. P., Sparling, J., & Miller-Johnson, S. (2002). Early childhood education: Young adult outcomes from the Abecedarian Project. *Applied Developmental Science, 6*, 42–57.

Cattell, P. (1940). *Cattell infant intelligence scale*. Psychological Corporation.

Center on the Developing Child at Harvard University. (2008). In Brief: The science of early childhood development. Retrieved November 16, 2024 from http://developingchild.harvard.edu/download_file/-/view/64/3.

Center on the Developing Child at Harvard University. (2010). The foundations of lifelong health are built in early childhood. Retrieved November 16, 2024 from http://developingchild.harvard.edu/library/reports_and_working_papers/foundations-of-lifelong-health/.

Cesario, J., Johnson, D. J., & Eisthen, H. L. (2020). Your brain is not an onion with a tiny reptile inside. *Current Directions in Psychological Science: A Journal of the American Psychological Society, 29*(3), 255–260. https://doi.org/10.1177/0963721420917687

Chen, X. (2012). Culture, peer interaction, and socioemotional development. *Child Development Perspectives, 6*(1), 27–34.

Cole, B., Pickard, K., & Stredler-Brown, A. (2019). Report on the use of telehealth in early intervention in Colorado: Strengths and challenges with telehealth as a service delivery method. *International Journal of Telerehabilitation, 11*(1), 33–40. https://doi.org/10.5195/ijt.2019.6273

Collins, W. A., Maccoby, E. E., Steinberg, L., Hetherington, E. M., & Bornstein, M. H. (2000). Contemporary research on parenting: The case for nature and nurture. *The American Psychologist, 55*(2), 218–232. https://doi.org/10.1037/0003-066X.55.2.218

Danaher, J. (2011). Eligibility and policies and practice for young children under part B of IDEA. Retrieved from http://ectacenter.org/~pdfs/pubs/nnotes27.pdf.

Davis-Kean, P. E., Tighe, L. A., & Waters, N. E. (2021). The role of parent educational attainment in parenting and children's development. *Current Directions in Psychological Science, 30*(2), 186–192.

DiPietro, J. A. (2000). Baby and the brain: Advances in child development. *Annual Review of Public Health, 21*(1), 455–471. https://doi.org/10.1146/annurev.publhealth.21.1.455

Division for Early Childhood of the Council for Exceptional Children. (2014). Official DEC recommended practices, 2014. Retrieved November 16, 2024 from https://divisionearlychildhood.egnyte.com/dl/tgv6GUXhVo.

Early Childhood Technical Assistance Center (ECTA). (2024, September 9). Part C National Program Data. Retrieved November 16, 2024 from https://ectacenter.org/partc/partcdata.asp

Education for All Handicapped Children Act. 20 U.S.C. § 1401 (1975).

Education of the Handicapped Act Amendments of 1986. Pub. L. No. 99-457, 20 U.S.C. § 1470 (1986).

Evans, G. W. (2004). The environment of childhood poverty. *American Psychologist, 59*(2), 77–92.

Evans, G. W. (2021). The physical context of child development. *Current Directions in Psychological Science, 30*(1), 41–48.

Evans, G. W., & Cassells, R. C. (2014). Childhood poverty, cumulative risk exposure, and mental health in merging adults. *Clinical Psychological Science, 2*(3), 287–296. https://doi.org/10.1177/2167702613501496

Evans, G. W., & Kim, P. (2013). Childhood poverty, chronic stress, self-regulation, and coping. *Child Development Perspectives, 7*(1), 43–48.

Evans, G. W., Li, D., & Whipple, S. S. (2013). Cumulative risk and child development. *Psychological Bulletin, 139*(6), 1342.

Every Student Succeeds Act, 20 U.S.C. § 6301 (2015). Retrieved from https://www.congress.gov/bill/114th-congress/senate-bill/1177.

Feldman, R. S. (2019). *Development across the life span* (9th ed.). Pearson Education, Inc.

Fernald, L. C., Kariger, P., Engle, P., & Raikes, A. (2009). *Examining early child development in low-income countries: A toolkit for the assessment of children in the first five years of life.* World Bank.

Frankenhuis, W. E., & Nettle, D. (2020). The strengths of people in poverty. *Current Directions in Psychological Science, 29*(1), 16–21. https://doi.org/10.1177/0963721419881154

Frye, W. S., Gardner, L., Campbell, J. M., & Katzenstein, J. M. (2022). Implementation of telehealth during COVID-19: Implications for providing behavioral health services to pediatric patients. *Journal of Child Health Care, 26*(2), 172–184. https://doi.org/10.1177/13674935211007329

Gesell, A. (1925). *Gesell developmental schedules.* Stoelting.

Glynn, L. M., & Sandman, C. A. (2011). Prenatal origins of neurological development: A critical period for fetus and mother. *Current Directions in Psychological Science, 20*(6), 384–389.

Goodman, J. F. (1990). Infant intelligence: Do we, can we, should we assess it? In C. R. Reynolds & R. W. Kamphaus (Eds.), *Handbook of psychological and educational assessment* (pp. 183–204). Guilford Press.

Griffiths, R. (1951). *The Griffiths mental development scale for testing babies from birth to two years.* Child Development Research Centre.

Guralnick, M. J. (1997). *The effectiveness of early intervention.* P.H. Brookes.

Hanna, J., Nickerson, G., & Pugliese E. (Executive Producers). (2007–2020). *Jack Hanna's Into the Wild* [TV Series]. Remedy Television and Branded.

Harlow, H. F. (1958). The nature of love. *The American Psychologist, 13*(12), 673–685. https://doi.org/10.1037/h0047884

Harris, J. R. (2000). Socialization, personality development, and the child's environments: Comment on Vandell (2000). *Developmental Psychology, 36*(6), 711–723. https://doi.org/10.1037/0012-1649.36.6.711

Hebbeler, K., Spiker, D., Bailey, D., Scarborough, A., Mallik, S., Simeonsson, R., & Singer, M. (2007). *Early intervention for infants & toddlers with disabilities and their families: participants, services, and outcomes. Final report of the National Early Intervention Longitudinal Study (NEILS).* SRI International.

Hughes, T. L., & Quinn, C. V. (2020). Working with young children living in stressful environments. In V. C. Alfonso & G. J. DuPaul (Eds.), *Healthy development in young children: Evidence-based interventions for early education* (pp. 297–315). American Psychological Association. https://doi.org/10.1037/0000197-015

Individuals with Disabilities Education Improvement Act [IDEA] of 2004, 20 U.S.C 1400 et seq. (2004).

Jacquet, L. (Director). (2005). *March of the Penguins* [Film]. National Geographic; Boone Pioche; Wild Bunch.

Karoly, L. A., Kilburn, M. R., Bigelow, J. H., Caulkins, J. P., Cannon, J. S., & Chiesa, J. R. (2001). Assessing costs and benefits of early childhood intervention programs: Overview and application of the Starting Early Starting Smart Program. Seattle: Casey Family Programs; Santa Monica: RAND.

Karoly, L. A., Kilburn, M. R., & Cannon, J. S. (2005). *Early childhood interventions: Proven results, future promise.* RAND Corporation.

Kelley, M. F., & Surbeck, E. (2007). History of preschool assessment. In B. A. Bracken & R. Nagle (Eds.), *Psychoeducational assessment of preschool children* (4th ed., pp. 3–28). Lawrence Erlbaum Associates Publishers.

Kelly-Vance, L., & Ryalls, B. O. (2020). Play-based approaches to preschool assessment. In V. C. Alfonso, B. B. Bracken, & R. J. Nagle (Eds.), *Psychoeducational assessment of preschool children* (5th ed.). Routledge. https://doi.org/10.4324/9780429054099

Koger, S. M., Schettler, T., & Weiss, B. (2005). Environmental toxicants and developmental disabilities: A challenge for psychologists. *American Psychologist, 60*(3), 243.

Lee, D. K., Cole, W. G., Golenia, L., & Adolph, K. E. (2018). The cost of simplifying complex developmental phenomena: A new perspective on learning to walk. *Developmental Science, 21*(4), e12615. https://doi.org/10.1111/desc.12615

Litt, J. S., Glymour, M. M., Hauser-Cram, P., Hehir, T., & McCormick, M. C. (2018). Early intervention services improve school-age functional outcome among neonatal intensive care unit graduates. *Academic Pediatrics, 18*(4), 468–474. https://doi.org/10.1016/j.acap.2017.07.011

Locke, J. (1690/1947). *An essay concerning human understanding.* E. P. Dutton.

Maholmes, V., & King, R. B. (2012). *The Oxford handbook of poverty and child development.* Oxford University Publishing.

Mayer, M. (2002). Grandparents rearing grandchildren: Circumstances and interventions. *School Psychology International, 23*(4), 371–385. https://doi.org/10.1177/0143034302234001

McBride, G. M., Dumont, R., & Willis, J. O. (2011). *Essentials of IDEA for assessment professionals.* John Wiley & Sons.

McCloskey, G., Petry, B., McIntosh, L., Kelly, J., & Filacheck, J. (2020). Neuropsychological assessment of preschool children. In V. C. Alfonso, B. B. Bracken, & R. J. Nagle (Eds.), *Psychoeducational assessment of preschool children* (5th ed., pp. 375–398). Routledge. https://doi.org/10.4324/9780429054099

McLoyd, V. C. (1998). Socioeconomic disadvantage and child development. *The American Psychologist, 53*(2), 185–204. https://doi.org/10.1037/0003-066X.53.2.185

McWilliam, R. (2016). Birth to three: Early intervention. In B. Reichow, et al. (Eds.), *Handbook of early childhood special education* (pp. 75–84). Springer International Publishing.

Meadan, H., & Daczewitz, M. E. (2015). Internet-based intervention training for parents of young children with disabilities: A promising service-delivery model. *Early Child Development and Care, 185*(1), 155–169.

Morris, D. (1967). *The naked ape: A zoologist's study of the human animal.* McGraw-Hill.

Nagle, R. J., Gagnon, S. G., & Kidder-Ashley, P. (2020). Issues in preschool assessment. In V. C. Alfonso, B. B. Bracken, & R. J. Nagle (Eds.), *Psychoeducational assessment of preschool children* (5th ed., pp. 29–48). Routledge.

National Academies of Sciences, Engineering, and Medicine. (2016). Policies and practices for supporting family caregivers working in sciences, engineering, and medicine. Retrieved November 16, 2024 from: https://www.nationalacademies.org/our-work/policies-and-practices-for-supporting-family-caregivers-working-in-science-engineering-and-medicine.

National Association for the Education of Young Children. (2020). Developmentally appropriate practice position statement. Retrieved November 16, 2024 from https://www.naeyc.org/resources/position-statements/dap/contents.

National Association of School Psychologists. (2015). *Early childhood services: Promoting positive outcomes for young children [Position statement].* Author.

National Early Childhood Technical Assistance Center [NECTAC]. (2011). The importance of early intervention for infants and toddlers with disabilities and their families. Retrieved from https://ectacenter.org/~pdfs/pubs/importanceofearlyintervention.pdf.

No Child Left Behind Act of 2001. 20 U.S.C. § 6301 (2001).

Noyes-Grosser, D. M., Elbaum, B., Wu, Y., Siegenthaler, K. M., Cavalari, R. S., Gillis, J. M., & Romanczyk, R. G. (2018). Early intervention outcomes for toddlers with autism spectrum disorder and their families. *Infants and Young Children, 31*(3), 177–199. https://doi.org/10.1097/IYC.0000000000000121

Ore, T. (2021). How effective is the use of telehealth for children with autism spectrum disorders. *International Journal of Psychiatry Research, 4*(1), 1–4.

Penney, C., & Scott, M. (Executive Producers). (2019 – present). *Earth Odyssey with Dylan Dreyer* [TV Series]. National Broadcasting Company.

Perone, S., Simmering, V. R., & Buss, A. T. (2021). A dynamical reconceptualization of executive-function development. *Perspectives on Psychological Science, 16*(6), 1198–1208.

Pinker, S. (2002). *The blank slate: The modern denial of human nature.* Viking.

Raines, T. C., Malone, C. M., Beidleman, L. M., & Bowman, N. (2020). National policies and laws affecting children's health and education. In V. C. Alfonso & G. J. DuPaul (Eds.), *Healthy development in young children: Evidence-based interventions for early education* (pp. 319–335). American Psychological Association. https://doi.org/10.1037/0000197-016

Ramey, C. T., Bryant, D. M., Sparling, J. J., & Wasik, B. H. (1985). Project CARE: A comparison of two early intervention strategies to prevent retarded development. *Topics in Early Childhood Special Education, 5,* 12–25.

Ramey, C. T., & Campbell, F. A. (1984). Preventive education for high-risk children: Cognitive consequences of the Carolina Abecedarian Project. *American Journal of Mental Deficiency, 88,* 515–523.

Ramey, C. T., Collier, A. M., Sparling, J. J., Loda, R. A., Campbell, F. A., Ingram, D. L., & Finkelstein, N. W. (1976). The Carolina Abecedarian Project: A longitudinal and multidisciplinary approach to the prevention of developmental retardation. In T. D. Tjossem (Ed.), *Intervention strategies for high risk infants and young children* (pp. 629–665). University Park Press.

Ramey, C. T., McGinness, G., Cross, L., Collier, A., & Barrie-Blackley, S. (1981). The Abecedarian approach to social competence: Cognitive and linguistic intervention for disadvantaged preschoolers. In K. Borman (Ed.), *The social life of children in a changing society* (pp. 145–174). Erlbaum Associates.

Ramey, C. T., & Ramey, S. L. (1998). Prevention of intellectual disabilities: Early interventions to improve cognitive development. *Preventive Medicine, 27,* 1–9.

Ramey, C. T., & Ramey, S. L. (1999). *Right from birth: Building your child's foundation for life.* Goddard Press.

Ramey, C. T., & Ramey, S. L. (2004). Early learning and school readiness: Can early intervention make a difference? *Merrill-Palmer Quarterly, 50*(4), 471–491. https://doi.org/10.1353/mpq.2004.0034

Ramey, C. T., Sparling, J. J., & Ramey, S. L. (2012). *Abecedarian: The ideas, the approach, and the findings.* Sociometrics.

Ramey, C. T., Sparling, J. J., & Ramey, S. L. (2014). Interventions for students from impoverished environments. In J. T. Mascolo, V. C. Alfonso, & D. P. Flanagan (Eds.), *Essentials of planning, selecting and tailoring interventions for unique learners* (pp. 415–448). John Wiley & Sons.

Redden, S. C., Forness, S. R., Ramey, S. L., Ramey, C. T., Brezausek, C. M., & Kavale, K. A. (2001). Children at risk: Effects of a four-year Head Start transition program on special education identification. *Journal of Child and Family Studies, 10,* 255–270.

Redden, S. C., Forness, S. R., Ramey, S. L., Ramey, C. T., Zima, B. T., Brezausek, C. M., & Kavale, K. A. (1999). Head Start children at third grade: Preliminary special education identification and placement of children with emotional, learning, and related disabilities. *Journal of Child and Family Studies, 8,* 285–303.

Reid, V. M., & Dunn, K. (2021). The fetal origins of human psychological development. *Current Directions in Psychological Science, 30*(2), 144–150. https://doi.org/10.1177/0963721420984419

Romeo, R. R., Leonard, J. A., Robinson, S. T., West, M. R., Mackey, A. P., Rowe, M. L., & Gabrieli, J. D. E. (2018). Beyond the 30-million-word gap: Children's conversational exposure is associated with language-related brain function. *Psychological Science, 29*(5), 700–710. https://doi.org/10.1177/0956797617742725

Rosenberg, S., Zhang, D., & Robinson, C. (2008). Prevalence of developmental delays and participation in early intervention services for young children. *Pediatrics, 121*(6), e1503–e1509. https://doi.org/10.1542/peds.2007-1680

Sattler, J. M. (2018). *Assessment of children: Cognitive foundations and applications* (6th ed.). Jerome M. Sattler.

Schweinhart, L. J., Montie, J., Xiang, Z., Barnett, W. S., Belfield, C. R., & Nores, M. (2005). Lifetime effects: The High/Scope Perry Preschool study through age 40. *Monographs of the High/Scope Educational Research Foundation, 14*(3/4), 194–215. https://doi. org/10.1080/09500790008666969

Schweinhart, L. J., & Weikart, D. P. (1998). Why curriculum matters in early childhood education. *Educational Leadership, 55*(6), 57–60.

Snow, C., & Van Hemel, S. (2008). *Early childhood assessment: Why, what, and how.* National Academies Press.

Sutherland, R., Trembath, D., & Roberts, J. (2018). Telehealth and autism: A systematic search and review of the literature. *International Journal of Speech-Language Pathology, 20*(3), 324–336.

The World Bank. (2015). Annual Report 2015. Retrieved from https://documents.worldbank. org/en/publication/documents-reports/documentdetail/880681467998200702/ world-bank-annual-report-2015.

Trohanis, P. L. (2008). Progress in providing services to young children with special needs and their families: An overview to and update on the implementation of the Individuals with Disabilities Education Act (IDEA). *Journal of Early Intervention, 30*(2), 140–151.

Twardzik, E., Cotto-Negron, C., & MacDonald, M. (2017). Factors related to early intervention Part C enrollment: A systematic review. *Disability and Health Journal, 10*(4), 467–474.

U.S. Department of Education. (2020a, June 24). *OSEP fast facts: Infants and toddlers with disabilities.* Individuals with Disabilities Act. Retrieved November 16, 2024 from https:// sites.ed.gov/idea/osep-fast-facts-infants-and-toddlers-with-disabilities-20/.

U.S. Department of Education. (2020b, October 16). *OSEP fast facts: Children 3 through 5 served under part B, section 619 of the IDEA.* Individuals with Disabilities Education Act. Retrieved November 16, 2024 from https://sites.ed.gov/idea/osep-fast-facts-children-3-5-20.

United Nations Children Fund. (2017). *Early moments matter for every child.* Retrieved November 16, 2024 from https://www.unicef.org/media/files/UNICEF_Early_ Moments_Matter_for_Every_Child_report.pdf.

Vergunst, F., & Berry, H. L. (2022). Climate change and children's mental Health: A developmental perspective. *Clinical Psychological Science, 10*(4), 767–785.

Weikart, D. P. (1967). *Preschool intervention: A preliminary report of the Perry Preschool Project.* Campus Publishers.

Weikart, D. P. (1970). *Longitudinal results of the Ypsilanti Perry Preschool Project.* High/Scope Educational Research Foundation.

Wilder, S. (2014). Effects of parental involvement on academic achievement: A meta-synthesis. *Educational Review, 66*(3), 377–397. https://doi.org/10.1080/00131911.2013. 780009

World Health Organization. (2016) *International classification of diseases, tenth edition.* Retrieved from https://icd.who.int/browse10/2016/en.

Zigler, E. F., & Muenchow, S. (1992). *Head Start: The inside story of America's most successful educational experiment.* Basic Books.

ANNOTATED BIBLIOGRAPHY

Alfonso, V. C., Bracken, B. A., & Nagle, R. J. (Eds.). (2020). *Psychoeducational assessment of preschool children* (5th ed). Routledge

The fifth edition of this seminal edited text on the assessment of preschoolers focuses on theory, research, and application. Chapters were written by expert researchers and practitioners who emphasized the importance of ecological assessment. Practitioners can gain in-depth knowledge about the assessment of cognitive, language, motor, social–emotional, play, and many other domains of functioning.

Alfonso, V. C., & DuPaul, G. J. (Eds.). (2020). *Healthy development in young children: Evidence-based interventions for early education.* American Psychological Association

This edited volume brings together a thorough collection of invited chapters by renowned researchers and practitioners in early childhood assessment, intervention, and advocacy. Topics include, among others, early childhood assessment, preparing children for successful school experiences, and creating learning environment that promote academic and social success and encourage creativity, as well as discussion of policies and laws that affect the health and education of young children. Chapters are also provided on special populations, including those with disabilities, those who come from linguistically and culturally diverse backgrounds, and those living in stressful environments.

Graves, S. L., & Blake, J. J. (2016). *Psychoeducational assessment and intervention for ethnic minority children: Evidence-based approaches.* American Psychological Association

This comprehensive resource is written for those practitioners who are seeking information on the psychoeducational assessment of and interventions for ethnic minority children. Although the book focuses on ethnic minority children of all ages, there is a chapter specifically on early childhood assessment for diverse learners. The volume is suitable for practitioners, researchers, and graduate students.

Grigorenko, E. (2009). *Multicultural psychoeducational assessment.* Springer.

This edited volume includes an examination and discussions of how different cultures measure intelligence and skill as well as why they use the tools they use. In addition, how their assessment methods are changing in the globalizing world is covered. Each contributor discusses how methods of assessment are limited and culture-bound and thus must be revised and adapted to other cultures.

Snow, C., & Van Hemel, S. (2008). *Early childhood assessment: Why, what, and how.* National Academies Press.

This text on assessment provides information about programs developed to enhance the school readiness of all young children, especially those from low-resource environments and communities and youth with disabilities. In addition, this volume affirms that assessments can make important contributions to the improvement of children's well-being when they are well-designed, implemented effectively, developed in the context of systematic planning, and are interpreted and used appropriately. Early Childhood Assessment addresses these characteristics by identifying important outcomes for children from birth to age 5 years and the quality and purposes of different techniques and instruments for developmental assessments.

ONLINE RESOURCES

Center for Response to Intervention in Early Childhood (CRTIEC): http://crtiec.org/. CRTIEC conducts research and provides resources that support application of Response to Intervention (RTI) in Early Childhood Education. In addition, it provides information about progress monitoring, evidence-based interventions, and current programs that implement RTI components in Early Childhood Education.

Division of Early Childhood (DEC): www.dec-sped.org/. The DEC advocates for policies and evidence-based practices that support families and enhance the highest-quality development of young children (0–8 years) who have or are at risk for developmental delays and disabilities.

It is an international membership organization for those who work with young children with disabilities as well as other needs.

Early Learning Guidelines (ELG) Educator Toolkit: www.apa.org/education/k12/ early-learning-guidelines. The ELG Educator Toolkit focuses on young children's learning using the domains from the Head Start framework that serve as a guide to early childhood educators seeking national and state resources that are founded on evidence-based practices. The ELG Educator Toolkit locates resources for working with special populations and links to states that received funding from the federal race-to-the-top early learning challenge grants, and are engaging in developing up-and-coming practices for working preschool-age children in early child programs.

National Association for the Education of Young Children (NAEYC): www.naeyc.org/. The NAEYC promotes learning for children from birth through 8 years of age by connecting practice, policy, and research, with the goal of helping the early childhood profession hold high standards and to be recognized as a key aspect of society.

National Association of School Psychologists (NASP): www. nasponline.org/. NASP represents the profession of school psychology by pushing forward effective practices to improve students' learning, behavior, and mental health, and by maintaining essential standards for practice.

National Education Association (NEA): www.nea.org/. The NEA is an organization committed to advancing the cause of public education by recommending free, quality kindergarten programs and mandatory full-day kindergarten. The NEA also advocates for free, quality universal pre-k, pre-k available for disadvantaged families, and dedicated funding for early childhood education.

National Head Start Association (NHSA): www.nhsa.org/. The NHSA is committed to giving every child, regardless of circumstances at birth, an opportunity to succeed in school and in life. The NHSA focuses on early learning innovation and offers a unique whole child/whole family program design with a delivery system that includes local programs, national standards, monitoring, professional development, and family engagement.

Zero to Three: www.zerotothree.org/. Zero to Three's mission is to ensure that all babies and toddlers have a positive start to life and reach their full potential. The organization provides helpful resources, tools, and policies for parents, professionals, and policymakers, taking a unique approach to child development by connecting those who can truly make a difference in the life of a child with the research they need.

Two

UNIQUE CONSIDERATIONS AND FACTORS IN ASSESSING AND EVALUATING YOUNG CHILDREN

Assessing and evaluating (i.e., interpreting) young children's (i.e., 0–60 months) performance are two of the most rewarding experiences for those who engage in working with them, but at the same time, are not without unique considerations, factors, and, at times, challenges (Alfonso et al., 2022; Snow & Van Hemel, 2008), which is the primary focus of this chapter. As noted by Alfonso, Ruby, et al. (2020) assessing and evaluating young children are very different than assessing and evaluating school-age children or adolescents. For example, many young children do not have sustained attention spans, can be awkward physically (e.g., gross motor functioning that is not coordinated), and have limited expressive language skills.

These characteristics are not problematic as they are typical of young children (Bergen & Woodin, 2011; Bracken & Theodore, 2020a; Brassard & Boehm, 2007; Fletcher, 2011; Sattler, 2018). Nevertheless, these characteristics and several others, along with unique considerations and factors, make assessing and evaluating young children challenging, requiring examiners to keep these variables in mind when working with them. This is especially pertinent during direct assessments such as when administering standardized, norm-referenced tests like the Bayley Scales of Infant and Toddler Development, Fourth Edition (Bayley-4; Alfonso et al., 2022; Aylward, 2020; Bayley & Aylward, 2019). Of course, examiners also administer rating scales, conduct interviews, and engage in behavioral

---

Essentials of Assessing Infants, Toddlers, and Preschoolers, First Edition.
Brittany A. Dale, Joseph R. Engler, and Vincent C. Alfonso.
© 2025 John Wiley & Sons, Inc. Published 2025 by John Wiley & Sons, Inc.

observations (see Alfonso, Engler, et al., 2020 and Hojnoski & Missall, 2020 for further discussion of assessment methods). However, these methods tend to be more straightforward and often involve working with adults in the young child's life (Bracken & Theodore, 2020a).

This chapter introduces readers to many considerations, factors, and characteristics of young children to bear in mind when assessing and evaluating them. These considerations and factors are grouped into three categories: logistical, examiner, and child. In addition, a section of this chapter covers the characteristics of young children. Each category and its characteristics are discussed in the context of how they may impact the young child's assessment or test performance. Finally, we provide a discussion, albeit brief, on quantitative and qualitative characteristics of standardized, norm-referenced tests as they continue to be used with young children (Benson et al., 2019; Oakland et al., 2016), even though some scholars question or do not support this method of assessment (e.g., Bagnato & Neisworth, 1994; Goodman, 1990; Lidz, 2002; Macy & Bagnato, 2013). Although each section of this chapter could very well be a chapter on its own, space limitations preclude in-depth discussions of all concepts and topics herein. Interested readers may find other sources helpful as they delve into the world of assessing and evaluating young children. Some of these sources include Alfonso et al. (2022), Alfonso, Bracken, et al. (2020), Alfonso and Flanagan (1999, 2009), Bracken and Theodore (2020a,b), Bradley-Johnson and Johnson (2007), Brassard and Boehm (2007), Engler and Alfonso (2020); Lidz (2002), Losardo and Notari-Syverson (2011), Mowder et al. (2009), Nuttall (1999), and Sattler (2018).

LOGISTICAL CONSIDERATIONS AND FACTORS

There are a few critical logistical considerations and factors that can impact the young child's assessment or test performance as well as the examiner's evaluation of that performance. These include the assessment or testing location and materials, duration of the assessment or testing, and the presence of caregivers. Bracken and Theodore (2020b) discussed these at length; they are discussed briefly here and listed in Rapid Reference 2.1.

> ## ≋ Rapid Reference 2.1 Logistical Considerations and Factors That May Affect a Young Child's Performance
>
> - Assessment or testing location and materials
> - Duration of assessment or testing
> - Presence of caregivers

Assessment or Testing Location and Materials

Typically, when examiners are assessing or testing school-age children or adolescents, they do so in schools or other educational settings that may or may not be suitable for the activity depending on resources. Nevertheless, these activities take place primarily in schools and most likely do not include caregivers or other professionals in the room (Sattler, 2018). Although young children may be assessed or tested in various educational settings, it is not uncommon for them to take place in the child's home, the examiner's office, or a medical facility (Bayley & Aylward, 2019). These locations may or may not be familiar to the young child and thus can certainly affect performance. A rule of thumb in young children's assessment is to engage in a multi-source, multi-method, and multi-setting paradigm (Alfonso, Engler, et al., 2020). This paradigm assists in obtaining reliable and valid assessment data and evaluation of the young child as there should be ample data from which to draw conclusions and make data-based recommendations.

Bracken and Theodore (2020b) stated, "The effective assessment environment should be cheerful, convey safety, capitalize on the child's curiosity, and stimulate the child's participation. For a testing environment to do these things, it must be child-centered and friendly, and accommodate the needs of young children" (p. 66). Included in an effective assessment or testing environment are the furniture and table/chair arrangement, decorations, limited distractions, and climate control. For example, space for young children should include appropriately sized furniture that is comfortable and a table/chair arrangement that is conducive to engaging the young child and creating a safe assessment situation (Raiford & Coalson, 2014). It is not uncommon, however, for the assessment or testing to take place on the floor as that may be more comfortable and conducive for a reliable and valid assessment (Alfonso et al., 2005). For example, young children with physical challenges may be more comfortable on the floor (Sattler, 2018). Of course, the floor must be clean and if possible have carpeting that does not hamper the child's mobility.

In addition, assessment locations should be appealing with bright colored walls, toys, and other fun items for young children to assist with establishing and maintaining rapport (Bracken & Theodore, 2020b; Sattler, 2018). It is important, however, that assessment and testing locations are free from as many internal and external distractions as possible such as overly stimulating rooms or a location that is next to where there are many extraneous noises, respectively (Alfonso et al., 2022; Bayley & Aylward, 2019; Brassard & Boehm, 2007; Raiford & Coalson, 2014). Finally, the assessment or testing location should not be too hot or too cold as to interfere with the young child's performance or the examiner conducting a reliable and valid assessment. The temperature should be just right for the child and examiner.

Duration of the Assessment or Testing

Examiners must be aware of the young child's attention span, motivation, and any medical concerns when conducting the assessment or testing because these and other factors discussed later in this chapter may affect performance. All told, however, the direct, interactive assessment (i.e., testing) of young children should be kept to a time that ensures maximizing the validity of the results. This time (period) may range from as brief as 30 minutes to a longer time of 60 or more minutes depending on the child, materials used, and skillset of the examiner (Bayley & Aylward, 2019; Raiford & Coalson, 2014). Some measures for young children are highly engaging such as the Bayley-4 (Alfonso et al., 2022). An older test that is no longer used, but the genius creation of Dorothea McCarthy, the McCarthy Scales of Children's Abilities (MSCA; McCarthy, 1972) incorporated physical activity in the middle of the testing and at the same time assessed fine and gross motor functioning of the young child (Kaufman, 1977). Examiners should not be fearful of assessing or testing the young child over two or even three sessions as this may be necessary for some children and increase the validity of assessment results (Alfonso et al., 2005, 2022). Other methods of assessing young children such as rating scales or interviews with caregivers can take place at times other than the direct, interactive testing of the child.

Presence of Caregivers or Other Professionals

We believe that assessment or testing of young children should not be a mystery to their caregivers or other professionals working with them. It is critical that caregivers are included in the assessment and even present in the room where the assessment or testing takes place (Alfonso et al., 2005). This is somewhat different from decades ago when it was rare to have other adults in the room and from assessing or testing older children and adolescents, but it is essential when working with young children. For example, the Bayley-4 administration manual (Bayley & Aylward, 2019) explicitly states that caregivers should play a major role in the assessment of infants and toddlers, and we could not agree more. The presence of caregivers in the assessment room where testing is taking place serves the following purposes: (1) includes caregivers in the assessment process and helps establish rapport with the child and caregivers, (2) allows for engagement between the examiner and caregivers, (3) provides immediate feedback to caregivers regarding their child's performance, and (4) is the right thing to do (Alfonso et al., 2022).

> **DON'T FORGET 2.1**
>
> It is critical that caregivers are included in the assessment process and even present in the room where the assessment or testing is taking place.

If possible, it is beneficial to have one or two other professionals in the room or watching via a one-way mirror as this affords the other professionals the opportunity to hear and see the child engaging in the assessment process (Lidz, 2002; Linder, 2008; Losardo & Notari-Syverson, 2011). To do right by the child and the family, it is imperative that all professionals involved in the assessment process contribute their expertise to understand better the developing child. Assessing young children, especially those with developmental delays, is no easy task and all those involved in the child's life should play a role in assuring a healthy trajectory (Alfonso et al., 2024; Bayley & Aylward, 2019).

EXAMINER CONSIDERATIONS AND FACTORS

Like logistical considerations and factors that can impact the young child's performance as well influence the examiner's evaluation of performance, there are examiner considerations and factors. These include, but are not limited to, approachability/affect, physical presence, rapport, behavior management skills, psychometric skill, and experience with young children. As with logistical considerations and factors, Bracken and Theodore (2020b) discussed these at length. Here, they are discussed briefly and listed in Rapid Reference 2.2.

≡ Rapid Reference 2.2 Examiner Considerations and Factors That May Affect a Young Child's Performance

- Approachability/affect
- Physical presence
- Rapport
- Behavior management skills
- Psychometric skill
- Experience with young children

Approachability/Affect

Examiners must be approachable and express a warm, welcoming affective reception to the young child and caregivers (Alfonso et al., 2022; Bayley & Aylward, 2019; Raiford & Coalson, 2014). Young children *know* when they encounter adults who do not like them and are almost immediately *turned off* to the assessment process calling into question the validity of results. When instructing graduates students about assessing young children, we tell them not to work with young children if they do not like them because there is virtually no possibility of obtaining valid results (Ford et al., 2012). Young children typically want to do one thing: play. This desire is important to observe (e.g., Kelly-Vance & Ryalls, 2020; Lidz, 2002; Sahlberg & Doyle, 2019). Thus, the examiner must be playful and engage the young child as much as possible while conducting the assessment. How the examiner greets the child, engages with the child, and creates a warm, caring, and safe environment are critical in the assessment process as they can make or break the experience for the young child (Bracken & Theodore, 2020b; Raiford & Coalson, 2014; Sattler, 2018). In addition, given that other adults may be in the room, the examiner wants to demonstrate that he or she is approachable, playful, and at the same time professional (Lidz, 2002; Linder, 2008; Losardo & Notari-Syverson, 2011).

Physical Presence

The examiner must be well kempt while at the same time wear comfortable clothes and shoes as testing with young children oftentimes requires sitting on the floor or being very active (e.g., watching the child, navigating test materials, answering questions, etc.) (Alfonso et al., 2005, 2022; Ford et al., 2012; Raiford & Coalson, 2014). The third author of this volume assessed hundreds of young children and had to abandon the collared shirt and tie for jeans or casual pants, shirts, and shoes! That was smart as it is not uncommon when working with infants that there are various fluids with which the examiner may come into contact. Although not always pleasant, it is incumbent upon the examiner to treat mucous from runny noses, urine, and sweat during the assessment process as normal and typical of young children, especially those with developmental delays. Again, if one does not like young children, it is best not to work with them because more harm than good can be done.

> **DON'T FORGET 2.2**
>
> Although not always pleasant, it is incumbent upon the examiner to treat mucous from runny noses, urine, and sweat during the assessment process as normal and typical of young children, especially those with developmental delays.

Rapport

If the examiner cannot establish and maintain rapport with the young child (and adults in the room), the assessment results are not going to be reliable and valid (Ford et al., 2012; Raiford & Coalson, 2014). The primary goal of the examiner is to maximize the validity of the assessment or test results (Alfonso et al., 2022). The only way this can be accomplished is through having good, sustained rapport with the child. For the most part, young children really do not care what the examiner wants or that the examiner has a timeline to conduct the assessment or testing, evaluate performance, and write a report. That is not their concern or priority. As stated earlier, young children want to play, and the examiner is a new playmate. Thus, examiners should smile often, laugh appropriately, and reinforce young children's adaptive behavior (socially or via healthy edibles) (Alfonso et al., 2022).

Behavior Management Skills

One of the major points of this book and chapter is that assessing and evaluating young children is not the same as assessing and evaluating older children and adolescents (Ford et al., 2012). Examiners of young children must be able to navigate multiple variables during the assessment process, including managing the young child's behavior. This is no easy feat. Thus, examiners working with young children must have much energy, prior experience, education and training, and to some degree luck! According to Bracken and Theodore (2020a) "Examiners must know when and how to question, direct, cajole, tease, laugh, act silly, be stern, reinforce, admonish, talk, be quiet, pat the child's head or hand affectionately, slow down or speed up the administration pace, show genuine empathy, and perform a variety of related behaviors with perfect timing and sufficient sincerity to maintain the child's motivation, cooperation, and participation" (p. 65). This is a tall, but necessary order for examiners of young children.

Psychometric Skill and Experience with Young Children

Assessment of young children involves tools, instruments, or measures on which most examiners were not educated or trained (Alfonso, Ruby, et al., 2020). In-depth knowledge of these tools, instruments, and measures together with a fair amount of experience are required before beginning to assess young children. This is difficult to achieve as the assessment of young children continues to be inadequately addressed in graduate programs, internships, and the like (Alfonso et al. 2022; Schmitt et al., 2020). Although some standardized, norm-referenced tests are downward extensions of those designed for older children such as the Wechsler Preschool and Primary Scale of Intelligence-Fourth Edition (WPPSI-IV; Wechsler, 2012), most are not and require substantial understanding of and practice with administration, scoring, interpretation, and supervision. Examiners are advised to take courses, webinars, and other professional development experiences to master young child assessment (Alfonso, Ruby, et al., 2020; Ford et al., 2012). In addition, they need to be familiar with the quantitative and qualitative characteristics of these tools, instruments, and measures (Engler & Alfonso, 2020). These are addressed later in this chapter, but now we turn to child considerations and factors, and then characteristics of young children that deserve special attention.

CHILD CONSIDERATIONS AND FACTORS

Perhaps the most important considerations and factors to consider are those of the child who is being assessed. Knowledge of these considerations and factors along with experience are essential not only for the assessment of the child, but evaluation (i.e., interpretation of performance). Bracken and Theodore (2020a) caution that because observations of young children's behavior are not as reliable and valid as standardized, norm-referenced assessment (testing) considerable thought must be given to the impact these behaviors have on the examiner's evaluation of assessment and test performance. Nevertheless, observations of young children's behavior provide a clinically rich picture of young children and insights as to how their behavior affects their test and nontest performance (Bracken & Theodore, 2020a; Brassard & Boehm, 2007; Raiford & Coalson, 2014; Sattler, 2018). Finally, just as examiners must become skilled at administering, scoring, and interpreting test performance (APA, 2020), they must become skilled observers to increase the validity of their decisions.

> ## CAUTION 2.1
>
> Observations of young children's behavior are not as reliable and valid as standardized, norm-referenced assessment (testing); therefore, considerable thought must be given to the impact these behaviors have on the examiner's evaluation of assessment and test performance.

According to Bracken and Theodore (2020a) and Wright (2021), child considerations and factors are many such as appearance (including height and weight, physical abnormalities, grooming and dress), overall health, speech, fine and gross motor skills, and affect/mood. Table 2.1 lists these considerations and factors along with some comments regarding why they are important to note and the possible influence on assessment/test performance. Next, we address several characteristics of young children that deserve special attention and that novice young child examiners may not be mindful of on a regular basis.

Table 2.1 Child Considerations and Factors That May Affect Assessment/Test Performance

Child Consideration/ Factor	Comment
Appearance including height, weight, physical abnormalities, grooming, and dress	Examiners should observe the child's height and weight to determine if the child is within normal limits, overweight, or underweight. For example, a young child with obesity may encounter difficulties completing gross motor tasks. In addition, examiners should note any physical abnormalities that could indicate abuse or neglect. Finally, how a child is dressed and appears are important as a neatly groomed child in clean clothes is most likely coming from a different home environment than a child who is wearing dirty or torn clothes and is disheveled.
General Health	A young child's general health should be noted as a child who is often sick or who has not received a physical exam in a long time may not perform optimally. A young child who is healthy typically exhibits age-appropriate energy, motivation, and eagerness to play with the examiner and thus yield reliable and valid assessment or test results.
Speech	Examiners should listen carefully to the young child's speech for stuttering, stammering, or other speech anomalies (e.g., lisp). Observations of speech in the young child may "yield a great deal of information about not only the quality of the child's language skills but also the child's overall cognitive ability and level of social-emotional development" (Bracken & Theodore, 2020a, p. 44: Caesar & Ottley, 2020; Hoover et al., 2011; Sattler, 2018).
Fine and Gross Motor Skills	Whether assessing fine and gross motor skills formally or these skills are used in performing other tasks, examiners should note any motor difficulties or challenges (Monsma et al., 2020). Many young children from low-resourced environments may not have experiences with blocks, crayons, etc. and thus not perform as well as children from high-resourced environments (Hughes & Quinn, 2020). Low performance, therefore, may be due to lack of experience or exposure rather than lack of skill (Mendez & LaForrett, 2020). An adaptive behavior scale may be useful in gathering important data on the young child's motor functioning (Harrison, 2020).
Affect/Mood	Most young children are happy and find assessment or testing with an adult an enjoyable experience. Therefore, if a young child appears sad or cries during the assessment or testing, it is critical to note and try to understand why. A negative affective state can impede optimal functioning and should be noted (Whitcomb & Kemp, 2020). Interviewing the caregiver is essential to determine why the young child is not in a happy mood and interpret performance accordingly (Hojnoski & Missall, 2020).

CHARACTERISTICS OF YOUNG CHILDREN THAT DESERVE SPECIAL ATTENTION

Like young child considerations and factors that examiners should note during the assessment process, there are characteristics of young children that should be observed and integrated into the examiner's evaluation of the child. These include expressive and receptive language, activity level, attention span (distractibility and impulsivity), motivation, temperament, and cultural and linguistic diversity (Alfonso et al., 2022; Bayley & Aylward, 2019; Bracken & Theodore, 2020a; Brassard & Boehm, 2007; Lidz, 2002; Ortiz & Wong, 2020; Radzicki et al., 2020; Raiford & Coalson, 2014; Sattler, 2018). Each of these characteristics is discussed below and listed in Rapid Reference 2.3.

> ### ≡ Rapid Reference 2.3 Characteristics of Young Children That Deserve Special Attention
>
> - Expressive and receptive language skills
> - Activity level
> - Attention span (distractibility and impulsivity)
> - Motivation
> - Temperament
> - Cultural and linguistic diversity

Expressive and Receptive Language Skills

Many young children do not have highly developed expressive or receptive language skills. In fact, one of the most frequent reasons for referral is language delay. Typically, receptive language skills develop first followed by expressive language skills (Caesar & Ottley, 2020; Wiig, 2011). That is, young children understand language prior to expressing themselves verbally, but any pattern of development can occur. In addition, there is a close relationship between young children's cognitive and language development. For instance, many items on cognitive measures for young children assess language abilities (Raiford & Coalson, 2014). For example, the Bayley-4 assesses receptive and expressive language skills separately from cognitive skills, but there is some overlap (Alfonso et al. 2022; Aylward, 2020; Bayley & Aylward, 2019). Furthermore, many subtests within a test battery are not

CAUTION 2.2

When assessing developmental domains other than language, it is important not to penalize the young child for language because language is not the construct being assessed.

pure measures of a single skill. When assessing developmental domains other than language, it is important not to penalize the young child for language because language is not the construct being assessed (Bracken, 1986; Flanagan et al., 1995; Huk et al., 2021).

Examiners may want to consult excellent resources to learn more about young children's developing language skills and how to assess those skills. For example, Caesar and Ottley (2020) provide a thorough chapter on assessing communication, language, and speech in preschool children that includes a useful table on typical speech and language milestones. Brassard and Boehm (2007) also provide a good read on young children's developing language skills. Measures of young children's language such as the Clinical Evaluation of Language Fundamentals Preschool-Third Edition (CELF Preschool-3; Wiig et al., 2020) also address language development and interpretation of young children's performance. Finally, the Appendix in this volume lists multiple measures of young children's language, and Engler et al. (2022) provided a psychometric review of some of these preschool language tests.

Activity Level

Examiners who think that young children are going to sit still during an assessment as older children often do, may be very surprised to learn that many young children do not sit still. At the same time, some young children may be underactive, and others may be overactive. Thus, it is incumbent upon the examiner to allow the young child to be active and at the same time to ensure reliable and valid assessment or test results. As stated earlier, there are, and were, some measures that include the assessment of motor skills (e.g., Bayley-4, MSCA) and including the assessment of motor skills may be useful during the assessment of other developmental domains as it may calm down the overactive child or provide a needed break for the child and the examiner alike.

Examiners should inquire if a young child's activity level during the assessment is typical or atypical of the child by asking their caregiver. It is not uncommon for examiners to believe that an active young child may have attention deficit hyperactivity disorder, but this disorder should not be considered unless a thorough behavioral assessment is conducted with the appropriate psychometrically sound methods (e.g., rating, scales, observations, interviews) (Alfonso, Engler, et al., 2020; Goldstein et al., 2011; Miller et al., 2011; Terjesen et al., 2019).

Attention Span (Distractibility and Impulsivity)

Like activity level, examiners should not be surprised by encountering a young child who is distractible or impulsive as these characteristics are typical in young children (e.g., Smoller, 1985). In fact, it may be noteworthy if the child is too quiet, focused, or sedentary. Again, the examiner must ensure reliable and valid assessment or test results and thus must manage the young child's behavior as noted earlier in this chapter. Effectively, "The examiner should differentiate a child's failure due to inability and failure due to inconsistent attention" (Bracken & Theodore, 2020a, p. 49). If the young child is too distracted or impulsive on the day of the assessment or testing, it may be necessary to conduct the assessment or testing another day. This is a clinical judgment call, and experienced examiners typically make this call easily. Finally, sometimes the presence of a caregiver can facilitate the assessment or testing with the highly distracted or impulsive young child (e.g., Alfonso et al., 2022).

> **DON'T FORGET 2.3**
>
> If the young child is too distracted or impulsive on the day of the assessment or testing, it may be necessary to conduct the assessment or testing another day.

Motivation

As stated earlier, young children want to play and if they do not find the assessment or testing *playful,* they may not be motivated to engage with the examiner (Lidz, 2002; Sahlberg & Doyle). Measures used with young children such as the Bayley-4, WPPSI-IV, Battelle Developmental Inventory-Third Edition (BDI-3; Newborg, 2020), and others include appealing materials that motivate young children to *play* with examiners. However, motivation may wane at times. Physical activity, breaks, healthy edibles, and the like may keep the young child motivated.

Temperament

According to Bracken and Theodore (2020b), "Examiners can facilitate the assessment of preschool children if they accommodate the temperament styles of their examinees" (p. 61). In other words, the more the examiner knows about the young child to be assessed or tested, the better. Examiners should interview the primary caretakers to gather information regarding personality characteristics, activity level, attention span, motivation, speech and language quality, and likes and dislikes (Lidz, 2002; Sattler, 2018). The informed examiner has time to create an assessment or testing environment that is conducive to obtaining reliable and valid data rather than an environment that creates an unsavory or challenging environment.

Cultural and Linguistic Diversity

The number of young children in the United States who are culturally and linguistically diverse (CLD) is increasing each year. For example, Radzicki et al. (2020) wrote:

In 2018, 15.3% of students enrolled in school identified as African American, 27.5% as Hispanic, 5.6% as Asian/Pacific Islander, and 3.1% as two or more races (National Center for Education Statistics, 2018). Furthermore, 9.5% of students enrolled in public school in the United States in 2015 were described as English learners (National Center for Education Statistics, 2018), indicating that these children do not communicate fluently or learn effectively in English (Castro-Olivo et al., 2018). The United States Census Bureau (Vespa et al., 2018) predicted that by 2060, 17% of the population will be foreign-born. Additionally, the population of children who identify as two or more races is predicted to double from 5.3% to 11.3% by 2060.

Although this is a positive fact for the country, examiners may not be educated about or have experience with young children who are CLD, posing additional challenges to assessment and testing. Indeed, Ortiz and Wong (2020) stated, "Without understanding cultural and linguistic influences on child development, there can be little-to-no hope of ensuring fairness and equity for children from diverse backgrounds" (p. 347). Therefore, it is incumbent upon examiners to become familiar with topics such as developmental language proficiency, acculturative knowledge acquisition, and modified methods of assessment and evaluation, among others (Ortiz & Wong, 2020). Interested readers may want to consult Ortiz and Wong (2020),

Radzicki et al. (2020), Brassard and Boehm (2007), Sattler (2018), and Engler and Alfonso (2020) for detailed discussions on assessing young children who are CLD as well as how to use the Culture-Language Interpretive Matrix or C-LIM to assist in evaluation of young children's performance on standardized, norm-referenced cognitive ability tests (Cormier et al., 2014, 2022; Flanagan et al., 2013, 2017; Ortiz, 2019, 2024).

QUANTITATIVE AND QUALITATIVE CHARACTERISTICS OF MEASURES USED WITH YOUNG CHILDREN

Many examiners are not excited about the quantitative characteristics of the tools, instruments, and measures they use. Yet, these quantitative (and qualitative) characteristics are important to consider especially in evaluating young children's performance. Standardized, norm-referenced tests, rating scales, and other measures used with young children have been evaluated for their quantitative or psychometric properties for decades and some have been evaluated for their qualitative characteristics (e.g., Alfonso et al., 2022; Alfonso & Flanagan, 1999, 2009; Bracken, 1987; Engler & Alfonso, 2020; Floyd et al., 2015; Terjesen et al., 2019). Below is a brief explanation of the quantitative and qualitative characteristics we believe to be important as well as criteria for evaluating the quantitative characteristics. Examiners may use this information in selecting the best tests, scales, or other measures when working with young children (see the Appendix, this volume). Interested readers may find the *Standards for Educational and Psychological Testing* (American Educational Research Association [AERA], American Psychological Association [APA], & National Council on Measurement in Education [NCME], 2014), the National Association of School Psychologists (2015) position statement on early childhood services, and the APA's (2020) guidelines for psychological assessment and evaluation helpful as well.

QUANTITATIVE CHARACTERISTICS

The quantitative characteristics to be familiar with include standardization, reliability, floors and ceilings, and item gradients. In addition, the validity of test scores or performance is very important to consider. Table 2.2 provides the criteria for evaluating most of the quantitative characteristics of measures used with young children. Recently, Alfonso et al. (2022) used the criteria in Table 2.2 to evaluate the quantitative characteristics of the Bayley-4 and found that this seminal measure continues to be a gold standard in the field of infant and toddler assessment.

Table 2.2 Criteria for Evaluating the Adequacy of the Quantitative Characteristics of Early Childhood Measures

Psychometric Characteristic	Criteria	Evaluative Classification
Standardization[a]		
Size of normative group and number of participants at each age/grade interval	200 persons per each 1-year interval and at least 2,000 persons overall	Good
	100 persons per each 1-year interval and at least 1,000 persons overall	Adequate
	Neither criterion above is met	Inadequate
Recency of normative data	Collected in 2014 or later	Good
	Collected between 2004 and 2013	Adequate
	Collected in 2002 or earlier	Inadequate
Age divisions of norm tables	One to two months	Good
	Three to four months	Adequate
	Greater than four months	Inadequate
Match of the demographic characteristics of the normative group to the U.S. population	Normative group represents the U.S. population on five or more important demographic variables (e.g., gender, race) with SES included	Good
	Normative group represents the U.S. population on three or four important demographic variables with SES included	Adequate
Reliability	Neither criterion is met	Inadequate
Internal consistency reliability coefficient (subtests and composites)	Greater than or equal to 0.90 (≥ 0.90)	Good
	0.80–0.89	Adequate
	Less than 0.80 (<0.80)	Inadequate
Test-retest reliability coefficient (composites only)	Greater than or equal to 0.90 (≥ 0.90)	Good

Table 2.2 (Continued)

Psychometric Characteristic	Criteria	Evaluative Classification
	0.80–0.89	Adequate
	Less than 0.80 (<0.80)	Inadequate
Test-retest reliability coefficient (subtests only)	Greater than or equal to 0.80 (≥0.80)	Adequate
	Less than 0.80 (<0.80)	Inadequate
Test-retest sample		
Size and representativeness of test-retest sample	Sample contains at least 100 participants and represents the U.S. population on at least five or more demographic variables	Good
	Sample contains at least 50 participants and represents the U.S. population on three or four demographic variables	Adequate
	Neither criterion is met	Inadequate
Age range of the test-retest sample	Spans no more than a 1-year interval	Good
	Spans no more than 2 years	Adequate
	Spans more than 2 years or extends beyond the preschool age range (i.e., 2–5 years.), regardless of interval size	Inadequate
Length of test-retest interval[b]	Interval ≤3 months	Good
	Interval >3 and ≤6 months	Adequate
	Interval >6 months	Inadequate
Test Floors		
Subtests[c]	Raw score of 1 is associated with a standard score greater than 2 standard deviations below the normative mean	Adequate
	Raw score of 1 is associated with a standard score less than or equal to 2 standard deviations below the normative mean	Inadequate

(Continued)

Table 2.2 (Continued)

Psychometric Characteristic	Criteria	Evaluative Classification
Composites[d]	Composite standard score greater than 2 standard deviations below the normative mean	Adequate
	Composite standard score less than or equal to 2 standard deviations below the normative mean	Inadequate
Ceilings		
Subtests[e]	Highest raw score obtained is associate with a standard score greater than 2 standard deviations above the normative mean	Adequate
	Highest raw score is associated with a standard score less than or equal to 2 standard deviations above the normative mean	Inadequate
Composites[f]	Composite standard score greater than 2 standard deviations above the normative mean	Adequate
	Composite standard score less than or equal to 2	Inadequate
Item gradients[g]		
Item gradient violations	No item gradient violations occur *or* all item gradient violations are between 2 and 3 standard deviations below the normative mean *or* the total number of violations is <5% across the age range of the test	Good
	All item gradient violations occur between 1 and 3 standard deviations below the normative mean *or* the total number of violations is ≥5% ≤15% across the age range of the test	Adequate
	All or any portion of item gradient violations occur between the mean and 1 standard deviation below the normative mean *or* the total number of violations is >15% across the age range of the test	Inadequate

Table 2.2 (Continued)

Psychometric Characteristic	Criteria	Evaluative Classification
Validity[h]		
Presence and quality of specific forms of validity evidences	5 or 6 forms of validity evidence and the authors' evaluation of available data	Good
	4 forms of validity evidence and the authors' evaluation of available data	Adequate
	<4 forms of validity evidence and the authors' evaluation of available data	Inadequate

[a] An overall rating is obtained as follows: Good = All Goods; Adequate = Goods and Adequates; Inadequate = Goods and/or Adequates, and Inadequates.

[b] The criteria presented here regarding the length of the test-retest interval differ from traditional criteria used with school-age children because young children's abilities change rapidly.

[c] Assuming a scale having a mean of 100 and a standard deviation of 15, a raw score of 1 that is associated with a standard score of ≤ 69 would constitute an adequate floor.

[d] Floors are calculated based on the aggregate of the subtest raw scores that comprise the composites, where one item per subtest is scored correctly.

[e] Assuming a scale having a mean of 100 and a standard deviation of 15, the highest raw score possible is associated with a standard score ≥ 131 would constitute an adequate ceiling.

[f] Ceilings are calculated based on the aggregate of the subtest raw scores that comprise the composites, where all items in a subtest are scored correctly.

[g] An item gradient is defined as the increase in standard score points associated with a one-point increase in raw score values. An item gradient violation occurs when a one-point increase in raw score points is associated with a standard score increase of greater than one third of a standard deviation (Bracken, 1987).

[h] The standards for validity in the 2014 publication *Standards for Educational and Psychological Testing* differ from those in the 1999 publication of the same name. Most notably, in the 2014 publication there is one overarching standard or guiding principle for validity with 25 standards subsumed under three clusters. The third cluster, namely, Specific Forms of Validity Evidence has 15 of the 25 standards subsumed under 6 forms of validity evidence. These 6 forms of validity evidence are akin to the 5 sources of validity evidence found in the 1999 publication and in earlier versions of this table. Ratings of "Good" or "Adequate" were made only when the available validity evidence was reviewed positively by the authors and corroborated by other reviews in the extant literature.

Standardization

A representative standardization sample allows examiners to determine the functioning of the young children they assess relative to the population at large (Sattler, 2018; Urbina, 2014). Typically, the standardization characteristics to evaluate include the size of the normative group, recency of normative data, age division of norm tables, and the match of the demographic characteristics of the normative group when compared to the United States population (see Alfonso & Flanagan, 1999, 2009; Engler & Alfonso, 2020 for detailed information). "Collectively, these standardization characteristics provide critical information regarding examiners' ability to generalize assessment results" (Alfonso et al., 2022, p. 208).

Reliability

If test scores are not reliable, they cannot be valid as reliability sets the ceiling on validity (Urbina, 2014). Typically, we think of *evidences* of reliability including internal consistency, test–retest, and interrater reliability (AERA, APA, & NCME, 2014; APA, 2020; Brassard & Boehm, 2007). Each offers evidence not only for the reliability of test scores, but also for the validity of test scores. Internal consistency reliability indicates the amount of confidence we have in the construct we are measuring, that is, the higher the reliability, the less measurement error and thus increased confidence. Test–retest reliability refers to stability over time and typically is assessed via testing a portion of the standardization sample two times after an intervening period of time (i.e., test–retest sample). Table 2.2 includes criteria for evaluating several characteristics of the test–retest sample. Finally, interrater reliability pertains to the consistency in ratings by different examiners or raters of a variable such as behavior observations of a child during an assessment.

Test Floors and Ceilings

Adequate test floors ensure that a young child's performance is not overestimated at the lower levels of ability or functioning. Effectively, test authors and publishers must include enough *easy* items to capture accurately those children who perform on the lower end of the normal ability continuum (Alfonso & Flanagan, 1999, 2009). An adequate test floor is obtained when a raw score of 1 is associated with a scaled or standard score greater than two standard deviations below the mean (see Alfonso & Flanagan, 1999, 2009; Bracken, 1987 for more details).

Adequate ceilings ensure that test performance is not underrepresented at the higher levels of functioning (Engler & Alfonso, 2020). An adequate ceiling is established when the highest obtained raw score is associated with a scaled or standard score greater than two standard deviations above the mean. Floors and ceilings apply to subtests and composites as noted in Table 2.2.

Item Gradients

Many examiners are not familiar with item gradients, but they are important, especially when assessing young children. Item gradients are associated with the incremental change in the conversion of raw scores to scaled or standard scores (Bracken & Theodore, 2020a). Item gradients are useful in differentiating young children's performance. There are a few ways in which to evaluate item gradients. For example, Bracken (1987) recommended that a raw score increase of 1 point should be associated with no greater than a 1/3 standard deviation difference. If an increase of greater than 1/3 standard deviation occurred, it would be considered an item gradient violation. Later, Alfonso and Flanagan (2009) provided guidance regarding the total number of item gradient violations within a test, suggesting that tests where no item gradient violations occur, or all item gradient violations occur between two and three standard deviations below the mean, or the total number of item gradient violations is less than 5% are good.

Validity

AERA et al. (2014) recommend that test authors and publishers provide validity evidence regarding test scores. The concept of validity is not easy to grasp and there have been myriad books and articles written on this psychometric characteristic over the past few decades (e.g., Kane, 2013; Lissitz, 2009; Markus & Borsboom, 2013). The complexity of validity, notwithstanding, examiners should be cognizant of test score validity by reviewing a test's technical manual. AERA et al. provide a good read on six validity *evidences* including content-oriented evidence, evidence regarding cognitive processes, evidence regarding internal structure, evidence regarding relationships with conceptually related constructs, evidence regarding relationships with criteria, and evidence based on consequences of tests. As written by several authors (e.g., Bracken, 1987; Flanagan & Alfonso, 1995), evidence of test score validity is not an all-or-nothing phenomenon and refers to several sources of evidence that support the interpretation of test scores (AERA et al., 2014; APA, 2020). As such, it is

> **DON'T FORGET 2.4**
>
> Evidence of test score validity is not an all-or-nothing phenomenon and refers to several sources of evidence that support the interpretation of test scores.

difficult to have criteria for which to evaluate validity. Table 2.2's evaluative criteria for validity include the presence of multiple *evidences* of validity in a test's manual and a review of that evidence and evidence found in the extant literature.

QUALITATIVE CHARACTERISTICS

In addition to being familiar with and evaluating the quantitative characteristics of a test, it is important to be familiar with the qualitative characteristics of the test. Indeed, Alfonso et al. (2022) wrote, "In some respects the qualitative characteristics of an instrument designed to assess young children's development are more important than the quantitative characteristics because it is incumbent upon the clinician to engage the young child for an extended period of time in order to obtain reliable and valid test performance results" (p. 35). Although evaluation of qualitative characteristics of tests has not received much attention in the literature, if at all, it is a necessary component of early childhood assessment as these characteristics impact test performance interpretation (i.e., evaluation). Alfonso and Flanagan (1999) provided a list and description of the qualitative characteristics they thought were important and these are provided in Rapid Reference 2.4. As these qualitative characteristics are more-or-less self-explanatory, they are not discussed here. Interested readers may find Alfonso and Flanagan's (1999) and Alfonso et al.'s (2022) explanations and applications of these important characteristics helpful.

Rapid Reference 2.4 Qualitative Characteristics of Early Childhood Measures

- Attractive Test Materials (e.g., manipulatives, colorful test materials)
- Efficient Administration Procedures (e.g., alternates verbal/nonverbal subtests, begins tasks with stimulating task)
- Expressive Language Requirement Unless Assessing Language (e.g., majority of tasks require one or two-word response, and/or gestures)
- Incorporates Nonverbal Score(s) Unless Assessing Language

- Limited Receptive Language Requirements Unless Assessing Language
- Directions are Suitable for Young Children
- Includes Opportunities to "Teach Task" (e.g., uses sample items, includes multiple trials, provides demonstrations)
- Includes Alternative Stopping Rules
- Translation or Adaptation Available in Other Languages
- Appropriate Degree of Language Demands and Cultural Loading

SUMMARY

Examiners who assess or test young children are fortunate as this work is highly rewarding, yet at the same time very challenging given many logistical, examiner, and child considerations and factors. This chapter touched upon these considerations and factors as well as the unique characteristics of young children. It is incumbent upon examiners who have limited to no experience working with young children to engage in professional development and supervision prior to assessing or testing them as the novice young child examiner may encounter situations that jeopardize the reliability and validity of the young child's performance. Even for experienced young child examiners, professional development and other activities would be helpful as technology, resources, and education are changing rapidly.

TEST YOURSELF

1. **Young children are different from school-age children and adolescents because typically they have:**
   (a) Limited expressive language skills
   (b) Shorter attention spans
   (c) Variable motivation
   (d) All of the above
2. **Considerations and factors to bear in mind when assessing and evaluating young children may be categorized as:**
   (a) Logistical
   (b) Examiner
   (c) A and B
   (d) None of the above

3. **The presence of caregivers during the assessment or testing of young children is:**
   (a) Frowned upon by most professionals
   (b) Supported by most professionals
   (c) Never permitted
   (d) Unethical

4. **Examiners working with young children should:**
   (a) Have experience working with this age group
   (b) Be patient, caring, and fun
   (c) Like young children
   (d) All of the above

5. **Quantitative characteristics of early childhood measures include the following except:**
   (a) Reliability
   (b) Standardization
   (c) Appealing test materials
   (d) Floors and ceilings

6. **Young children from low-resource environments:**
   (a) May not have experience with toys, technology, and other materials that young children from high-resource environments have
   (b) Are not as engaging as those from high-resource environments
   (c) Do not enjoy playing with adults
   (d) Do not perform well on early childhood measures

7. **Which of the following statements is true regarding assessing and evaluating young children:**
   (a) It is easier than assessing and evaluating school-age children
   (b) It takes less time than assessing and evaluating school-age children
   (c) It requires behavior management skills and knowledge of quantitative and qualitative characteristics of early childhood measures
   (d) None of the above

8. **Which of the following statements is false:**
   (a) Young children solely want to do what the examiner wants them to do
   (b) Young children want to play with the examiner
   (c) Caregivers can play a critical role in the assessment and evaluation of young children
   (d) Most examiners are not familiar with item gradients

9. If an early childhood measure is not reliable, it should not be:

    (a) Used with young children

    (b) Valid

    (c) Interpreted with confidence

    (d) All of the above

10. The main goal in assessing or testing young children is to:

    (a) Satisfy their parents curiosity about their functioning

    (b) Determine how to intervene with them, if necessary, to ensure a healthy life trajectory

    (c) Demonstrate the examiner's competence

    (d) Practice with early childhood measures

Answers: 1. d; 2. c; 3. b; 4. d; 5. c; 6. a; 7. c; 8. a; 9. d; 10. b

REFERENCES

Alfonso, V. C., Bracken, B. A., & Nagle, R. J. (2020). *Psychoeducational assessment of preschool children* (5th ed.). Routledge.

Alfonso, V. C., Engler, J. R., & Lepore, C. C. (2020). Assessing and evaluating young children: Developmental domains and methods. In V. C. Alfonso & G. J. DuPaul (Eds.), *Healthy development in young children: Evidence-based interventions for early education* (pp. 13–44). American Psychological Association.

Alfonso, V. C., Engler, J. R., & Stavrou, E. (2024). Assessment of preschoolers and school readiness. In L. A. Theodore, B. A. Bracken, & M. A. Bray (Eds.), *School psychology desk reference* (pp. 63–79). Oxford University Press.

Alfonso, V. C., Engler, J. R., & Turner, A. D. (2022). *Essentials of Bayley-4 assessment.* John Wiley & Sons.

Alfonso, V. C., & Flanagan, D. P. (1999). Assessment of cognitive functioning in preschoolers. In E. V. Nuttall, I. Romero, & J. Kalesnik (Eds.), *Assessing and screening preschoolers* (2nd ed., pp. 186–217). Allyn & Bacon.

Alfonso, V. C., & Flanagan, D. P. (2009). Assessment of preschool children: A framework for evaluating the adequacy of the technical characteristics of norm-referenced instruments. In B. Mowder, F. Rubinson, & A. Yasik (Eds.), *Evidence based practice in infant and early childhood psychology* (pp. 129–166). John Wiley & Sons.

Alfonso, V. C., Ruby, S., Wissel, A. M., & Davari, J. (2020). School psychologists in early childhood settings. In F. C. Worrell & T. L. Hughes (Eds.), *The Cambridge handbook of applied school psychology* (pp. 579–597). Cambridge University Press.

Alfonso, V. C., Russo, P. M., Fortugno, D. A., & Rader, D. E. (2005). Critical review of the Bayley scales of infant development (2nd ed.): Implications for assessing young children with developmental delays. *The School Psychologist, 59*(2), 67–73.

American Educational Research Association, American Psychological Association, & National Council on Measurement in Education. (2014). *Standards for educational and psychological testing.* American Educational Research Association.

American Psychological Association, APA Task Force on Psychological Assessment and Evaluation Guidelines. (2020). APA Guidelines for Psychological Assessment and Evaluation. Retrieved from https://www.apa.org/about/policy/guidelines-psychological-assessment-evaluation.pdf

Aylward, G. P. (2020). *Bayley 4 clinical use and interpretation*. Academic Press.

Bagnato, S. J., & Neisworth, J. T. (1994). A national study on the social and treatment invalidity of intelligence testing for early intervention. *School Psychology Quarterly, 9*, 81–102.

Bayley, N., & Aylward, G. P. (2019). *Bayley scales of infant and toddler development* (4th ed.). Pearson.

Benson, N., Floyd, R., Kranzler, J., Eckert, T., Fefer, S., & Morgan, G. (2019). Test use and assessment practices of school psychologists in the United States: Findings from the 2017 National Survey. *Journal of School Psychology, 72*, 29–48.

Bergen, D., & Woodin, M. (2011). Neuropsychological development of newborns, infants and toddlers (0 to 3 years old). In A. S. Davis (Ed.), *Handbook of pediatric neuropsychology* (pp. 15–30). Springer Publishing Company, LLC.

Bracken, B. A. (1986). Incidence of basic concepts in the directions of five commonly used American tests of intelligence. *School Psychology International, 7*, 1–10.

Bracken, B. A. (1987). Limitations of preschool instruments and standards for minimal levels of technical adequacy. *Journal of Psychoeducational Assessment, 5*, 313–326.

Bracken, B. A., & Theodore, L. A. (2020a). Observation of preschool children's assessment-related behaviors. In V. C. Alfonso, B. A. Bracken, & R. J. Nagle (Eds.), *Psychoeducational assessment of preschool children* (5th ed., pp. 32–54). Routledge.

Bracken, B. A., & Theodore, L. A. (2020b). Creating the optimal preschool testing situation. In V. C. Alfonso, B. A. Bracken, & R. J. Nagle (Eds.), *Psychoeducational assessment of preschool children* (5th ed., pp. 55–76). Routledge.

Bradley-Johnson, S., & Johnson, C. M. (2007). Infant and toddler cognitive assessment. In I. B. A. Bracken & R. J. Nagle (Eds.), *Psychoeducational assessment of preschool children* (4th ed., pp. 325–357). Lawrence Erlbaum Associates Publishers.

Brassard, M. R., & Boehm, A. E. (2007). *Preschool assessment: Principles and practices*. Guilford Press.

Caesar, L. G., & Ottley, S. W. (2020). Assessing communication, language, and speech in preschool children. In V. C. Alfonso, B. A. Bracken, & R. J. Nagle (Eds.), *Psychoeducational assessment of preschool children* (5th ed., pp. 250–282). Routledge.

Castro-Olivo, S. M., Preciado, J. A., Le, L., Marciante, M., & Garcia, M. (2018). The effects of culturally adapted version of *First Steps to Success* for Latino English language learners: Preliminary pilot study. *Psychology in the Schools, 55*, 36–49.

Cormier, D. C., Bulut, O., McGrew, K. S., & Kennedy, K. (2022). Linguistic influences on cognitive test performance: Examinee characteristics are more important than test characteristics. *Journal of Intelligence, 10*, 1–12.

Cormier, D. C., McGrew, K. S., & Ysseldyke, J. E. (2014). The influences of linguistic demand and cultural loading on cognitive test scores. *Journal of Psychoeducational Assessment, 32*, 610–623.

Engler, J. R., & Alfonso, V. C. (2020). Cognitive assessment of preschool children. In V. C. Alfonso, B. B. Bracken, & R. J. Nagle (Eds.), *Psychoeducational assessment of preschool children* (5th ed., pp. 226–249). Routledge.

Engler, J. R., Shanock, A., & Alfonso, V. C. (2022, April). *Examining the quantitative characteristics of preschool language tests: Implications for practice*. Roundtable presentation given at the annual meeting of the American Educational Research Association, San Diego, CA.

Flanagan, D. P., & Alfonso, V. C. (1995). A critical review of the technical characteristics of new and recently revised intelligence tests for preschool children. *Journal of Psychoeducational Assessment, 13*(1), 66–90.

Flanagan, D. P., Alfonso, V. C., Kaminer, T., & Rader, D. E. (1995). Incidence of basic concepts in the directions of new and recently revised intelligence tests for preschoolers. *School Psychology International, 16,* 345–364.

Flanagan, D. P., Ortiz, S. O., & Alfonso, V. C. (2013). *Essentials of cross-battery assessment* (3rd ed.). John Wiley & Sons.

Flanagan, D. P., Ortiz, S. O., & Alfonso, V. C. (2017). *Cross-battery assessment software system (X-BASS) (Version 2.0) [Computer software].* John Wiley & Sons.

Fletcher, K. L. (2011). Neuropsychology of early childhood (3 to 5 years). In A. S. Davis (Ed.), *Handbook of pediatric neuropsychology* (pp. 31–36). Springer Publishing Company, LLC.

Floyd, R. G., Shands, E. I., Alfonso, V. C., Phillips, J. F., Autry, B. K., Mosteller, J. A., Skinner, M., & Irby, S. (2015). A systematic review and psychometric evaluation of adaptive behavior scales and recommendations for practice. *Journal of Applied School Psychology, 31*(1), 83–113.

Ford, L., Kozey, M. L., & Negreiros, J. (2012). Cognitive assessment in early childhood: Theoretical and practical perspectives. In D. P. Flanagan & P. L. Harrison (Eds.), *Contemporary intellectual assessment: Theories, tests, and issues* (3rd ed., pp. 585–622). The Guilford Press.

Goldstein, S. J., Jansen, J., & Naglieri, J. A. (2011). Measurement of attention: Theoretical and operational considerations. In A. S. Davis (Ed.), *Handbook of pediatric neuropsychology* (pp. 251–260). Springer Publishing Company, LLC.

Goodman, J. F. (1990). Infant intelligence: Do we, can we, should we assess it? In C. R. Reynolds & R. W. Kamphaus (Eds.), *Handbook of psychological and educational assessment* (pp. 183–204). Guilford Press.

Harrison, P. L. (2020). Adaptive behavior assessment of preschool children. In V. C. Alfonso, B. A. Bracken, & R. J. Nagle (Eds.), *Psychoeducational assessment of preschool children* (5th ed., pp. 204–225). Routledge.

Hojnoski, R. L., & Missall, K. N. (2020). Considerations and methods in assessing early learning and social-emotional development in young children. In V. C. Alfonso & G. J. DuPaul (Eds.), *Healthy development in young children: Evidence-based interventions for early education* (pp. 297–315). American Psychological Association.

Hoover, J. R., Sterling, A. M., & Storkel, H. L. (2011). Speech and language development. In A. S. Davis (Ed.), *Handbook of pediatric neuropsychology* (pp. 71–78). Springer Publishing Company, LLC.

Hughes, T. L., & Quinn, C. V. (2020). Working with young children living in stressful environments. In V. C. Alfonso & G. J. DuPaul (Eds.), *Healthy development in young children: Evidence-based interventions for early education* (pp. 297–315). American Psychological Association.

Huk, O., Alfonso, V. C., & Le, K. (2021, February). *Presence of basic concepts in intelligence tests for preschool children.* Poster presented at the annual meeting of the National Association of School Psychologists, Baltimore, MD.

Kane, M. T. (2013). Validating the interpretations and uses of test scores. *Journal of Educational Measurement, 50,* 1–73.

Kaufman, A. S. (1977). *Clinical evaluation of young children with the McCarthy Scales.* Grune & Stratton.

Kelly-Vance, L., & Ryalls, B. O. (2020). Play-based approaches to preschool assessment. In V. C. Alfonso, B. B. Bracken, & R. J. Nagle (Eds.), *Psychoeducational assessment of preschool children* (5th ed., pp. 160–177). Routledge.

Lidz, C. S. (2002). *Early childhood assessment.* John Wiley & Sons.

Linder, T. W. (2008). *Transdisciplinary play-based assessment* (2nd ed.). Brookes Publishing.

Lissitz, R. W. (2009). *The concept of validity: Revisions, new directions, and applications.* IAP Information Age Publishing.

Losardo, A., & Notari-Syverson, A. (2011). *Alternative approaches to assessing young children* (2nd ed.). Paul H. Brookes Publishing Co.

Macy, M., & Bagnato, S. J. (2013). The authentic alternative for assessment in early childhood intervention. In D. H. Saklofske, C. R. Reynolds, & V. L. Schwean (Eds.), *The Oxford handbook of child psychological assessment* (pp. 671–682). Oxford University Press.

Markus, K. A., & Borsboom, D. (2013). *Frontiers of test validity theory: Measurement, causation, and meaning.* Routledge.

McCarthy, D. (1972). *The McCarthy scales of Children's Abilities.* Psychological Corporation.

Mendez, J., & LaForrett, D. (2020). Understanding the impact of poverty and implications for assessment with young children from low-resource backgrounds. In V. C. Alfonso, B. B. Bracken, & R. J. Nagle (Eds.), *Psychoeducational assessment of preschool children* (5th ed., pp. 399–420). Routledge.

Miller, M., Gelfand, J., & Hinshaw, S. P. (2011). Attention-deficit/hyperactivity disorder. In A. S. Davis (Ed.), *Handbook of pediatric neuropsychology* (pp. 565–580). Springer Publishing Company, LLC.

Monsma, E. V., Miedema, S. T., Brian, A. S., & Williams, H. G. (2020). Assessment of gross motor development in preschool children. In V. C. Alfonso, B. B. Bracken, & R. J. Nagle (Eds.), *Psychoeducational assessment of preschool children* (5th ed., pp. 283–319). Routledge.

Mowder, B. A., Rubinson, F., & Yasik, A. E. (2009). *Evidence-based practice in infant and early childhood psychology.* John Wiley & Sons.

National Association of School Psychologists. (2015). *Early childhood services: Promoting positive outcomes for young children [Position statement].* Author.

National Center for Education Statistics. (2018). Enrollment and percentage distribution of enrollment in public elementary and secondary schools, by race/ethnicity and level of education: Fall 1999 through fall 2027. Institute of Education Sciences. Retrieved from https://nces.ed.gov/programs/digest/d17/tables/dt17_203.60.as

Newborg, J. (2020). *Battelle developmental inventory* (3rd ed.). Riverside Insights.

Nuttall, E. V. E., Romero, I. E., & Kalesnik, J. E. (1999). *Assessing and screening preschoolers: Psychological and educational dimensions.* Allyn & Bacon.

Oakland, T., Douglas, S., & Kane, H. (2016). Top ten standardized tests used internationally with children and youth by school psychologists in 64 countries: A 24-year follow-up study. *Journal of Psychoeducational Assessment, 34,* 166–176.

Ortiz, S. O. (2019). On the measurement of cognitive abilities in English learners. *Contemporary School Psychology, 23,* 68–86.

Ortiz, S. O. (2024). The C-LIM Basic v6.1. Retrieved November 12, 2024 from http://facpub.stjohns.edu/~ortizs/CLIM/

Ortiz, S. O., & Wong, J. Y. T. (2020). Psychoeducational assessment of culturally and linguistically diverse preschool children. In V. C. Alfonso, B. B. Bracken, & R. J. Nagle (Eds.), *Psychoeducational assessment of preschool children* (5th ed., pp. 346–374). Routledge.

Radzicki, A., Hughes, T. L., Shoenenberger, A., Park, M., & Sanchez, Y. (2020). Working with young children who are culturally and linguistically diverse. In V. C. Alfonso & G. J. DuPaul (Eds.), *Healthy development in young children: Evidence-based interventions for early education* (pp. 275–295). American Psychological Association.

Raiford, S. E., & Coalson, D. L. (2014). *Essentials of WPPSI-IV assessment.* John Wiley and Sons.

Sahlberg, P., & Doyle, W. (2019). *Let the children play: How more play will save our schools and help children thrive.* Oxford University Press.

Sattler, J. M. (2018). *Assessment of children: Cognitive foundations and applications* (6th ed.). Jerome M. Sattler.

Schmitt, A., Wodrich, D. L., & Lorenzi-Quigley, L. (2020). Current status of pediatric topics in five school psychology journals: Publication trends between 2002 and 2019. *School Psychology, 35*(3), 171–178.

Smoller, J. W. (1985). The etiology and treatment of childhood. *Journal of Polymorphous Perversity, 2*, 3–7.

Snow, C. E., & Van Hemel, S. B. (2008). *Early childhood assessment: Why, what, and how.* National Academies Press.

Terjesen, M. D., Sciutto, M. J., & O'Brien, C. (2019). Behavior rating scales and the assessment of ADHD in early childhood: A review of psychometric properties and scale features. *Perspectives on Early Childhood Psychology and Education, 4*(1), 5–38.

Urbina, S. (2014). *Essentials of psychological testing* (2nd ed.). John Wiley and Sons.

Vespa, J., Armstrong, D. M., & Medina, L. (2018). Demographic turning points for the United States: Population projections for 2020 to 2060. *Current Population Reports* (No. P25-1144). Washington, DC: United States Census Bureau.

Wechsler, D. (2012). *Wechsler preschool and primary scale of intelligence* (4th ed.). Psychological Corporation.

Whitcomb, S. A., & Kemp, J. M. (2020). Behavior and socio-emotional skills assessment of preschool children. In V. C. Alfonso, B. B. Bracken, & R. J. Nagle (Eds.), *Psychoeducational assessment of preschool children* (5th ed., pp. 181–203). Routledge.

Wiig, E. H. (2011). Receptive and expressive language disorders in children. In A. S. Davis (Ed.), *Handbook of pediatric neuropsychology* (pp. 699–708). Springer Publishing Company, LLC.

Wiig, E. H., Secord, W. A., & Semel, E. (2020). *Clinical evaluation of language fundamentals preschool* (3rd ed.). Psychological Corporation.

Wright, A. J. (2021). *Conducting psychological assessment: A guide for practitioners* (2nd ed.). John Wiley & Sons, Inc.

Three

RESPONSIBLE ASSESSMENT OF YOUNG CHILDREN

According to Merriam-Webster (n.d.), the word *responsible* can be defined as "able to answer for one's conduct and obligations." When applied to the assessment of young children, responsible examiners should be able to articulate clearly and defend their choices within the assessment process, which includes the use of screening, progress monitoring, and diagnostic tools. That said, there is a dearth of literature related to young children that assists examiners in doing so (Schmitt et al., 2020). Therefore, this chapter provides a brief historical context and relevant literature that documents the importance of screening, progress monitoring, and diagnosis for young children. Then, we present and provide evaluative criteria regarding the most salient characteristics we believe examiners should consider when choosing diagnostic tools all while infusing unique differences between young children and other developmental ages (e.g., childhood, adolescence, and adulthood) into the discussion. The characteristics fall within the following broad categories: qualitative, quantitative, theoretical, and cultural/linguistic. We then summarize key takeaways examiners can use to gain confidence in their ability to articulate clearly and defend their choices within the assessment process.

HISTORICAL CONTEXT

The informal and formal assessment of young children dates back well over 100 years and includes several instrumental factors which have led to the increased importance of accurate assessment of young children (e.g., influential

Essentials of Assessing Infants, Toddlers, and Preschoolers, First Edition.
Brittany A. Dale, Joseph R. Engler, and Vincent C. Alfonso.
© 2025 John Wiley & Sons, Inc. Published 2025 by John Wiley & Sons, Inc.

figures, legislation, etc.). An in-depth discussion of all factors is excluded from this chapter due to space limitations (see Chapter 1, this volume for a more detailed discussion). That said, we focus the discussion on the importance of Head Start/ Early Head Start, the importance of the Education of All Handicapped Children Act of 1975, and the importance of Every Student Succeeds Act of 2015. In particular, we focus on how each relates to early childhood assessment.

Head Start/Early Head Start

On January 8, 1964, President Lyndon B. Johnson declared a "war on poverty" during his State of the Union address. The next year, the United States created an 8-week federally funded program called Project Head Start to help ameliorate the cycle of poverty that was affecting preschool-aged children. The original project was a comprehensive summer program that was designed for low-income families to address the social, emotional, nutritional, cognitive, and language needs of preschoolers through active parental involvement. Since its original inception, the program has continued to develop and now includes performance-based standards and is offered as a half-day or full-day option with year-round services. Consequently, young children in Head Start are supported to meet performance standards to improve school readiness (Office of Head Start, 2023).

In addition to Head Start, a federally funded program called Early Head Start was developed in 1995 to support pregnant mothers as well as children from birth to 3 years old. The Early Head Start Program has three different options for families: home-based support, center-based care, combination of home-based support, and center-based care. Similar in conception and operation to Head Start, the Early Head Start Program is committed to promoting healthy childhood development and preparing young children for success in school and beyond. Therefore, Head Start and Early Head Start agencies are responsible for assessing young children's developmental progression toward performance-based standards throughout their time in the program to promote future success.

Education for All Handicapped Children Act

Perhaps the most important legislation signed into law was the Education for All Handicapped Children Act (EHA) of 1975. The EHA provided a list of provisions that required a free and appropriate public education within the least restrictive environment to individuals with disabilities aged 5–21 years old throughout the United States. Under the EHA, all children with, or suspected with, a disability were entitled to a comprehensive evaluation at no cost to the parent(s). Therefore, school districts were required to develop evaluation procedures and protocols to identify school-aged children with disabilities and provide recommendations via an Individualized Education Program.

In 1986, the EHA was reauthorized. The reauthorized version of the EHA now included a provision for children birth to 3 years old. Prior to 1986, parents would have to wait until their child reached 3 years of age to be entitled to protections and services offered by the EHA. The 1986 reauthorization of the EHA brought a spotlight onto the importance of early identification of young children with disabilities and required states to begin identifying children with disabilities after they were born. In addition, the 1986 reauthorization of the EHA placed an increased emphasis on the importance of early intervention. In 1990, the EHA was reauthorized and its title changed to the Individuals with Disabilities Education Act (IDEA) of 1990. A year later, the classification of developmental delay was added to IDEA to serve children between 3 and 5 years old who are lagging behind their peers in one or more specific areas of development (e.g., cognitive, motor, language, etc.). Since then, eligibility under developmental delay has been extended to 9 years of age. The IDEA also included a separate section titled Part C, which focused on early intervention programs for infants and toddlers with disabilities. The subparts of the IDEA included general information as well as child find and assessment requirements. Infants and toddlers who were identified as having a disability were served on an Individualized Family Service Plan.

Every Student Succeeds Act

In 2015, Congress passed Every Student Succeeds Act (ESSA), which was a reauthorization of the No Child Left Behind Act of 2001. Although the primary focus of the ESSA is on elementary through high school education accountability standards, there are references that directly impact early childhood education. For example, the ESSA created a Preschool Development Grant Program for children birth to 5 years old (Office of Elementary & Secondary Education, 2023). The main purpose of the grant program is to help coordinate statewide needs assessments, develop strategic plans, and coordinate service delivery while increasing access to quality preschool programs (Alfonso et al., 2022). Consequently, the laws listed in the first section of this chapter have direct references to the assessment and identification of preschool-aged children. As a result of these laws, examiners should be familiar with the various types of assessment measures, including screening tools, progress monitoring tools, and diagnostic tools.

PRESCHOOL SCREENING

One way in which examiners can responsibly assess young children is by using screening tools. The overall purpose of screening young children is to identify whether they are "at-risk" of future difficulties. There are several appeals to using screening tools at the preschool level. First, screening tools are typically less expensive to purchase than their diagnostic counterparts. Therefore, from a financial perspective, screening tools provide more "bang for their buck" as higher percentages of young children can be assessed. Second, screening tools take significantly less time to administer than diagnostic tools. Consequently, examiner time may be utilized better by screening for developmental difficulties and/or delays. Third, screening tools can be used in group settings, whereas diagnostic tools are generally administered in a one-on-one setting. Fourth, a screening tool may identify a young child as being "at-risk" of developing a future problem and, therefore, may be entitled to early intervention services. This is especially relevant in organizations that use multitiered systems of support. A nonexhaustive list of advantages to using screening tools can be seen in Rapid Reference 3.1.

⪸ Rapid Reference 3.1 Advantages to Using Screening Tools

- Cost-effective
- Quick to administer
- Can be used in group settings
- Identifies young children as "at-risk" for developing future challenges

Although there are several advantages to screening young children, there are also disadvantages. Perhaps the most noticeable disadvantage is that screening tools typically have poorer psychometric properties than diagnostic tools. For example, screening tools generally have lower reliability coefficients and classification accuracy statistics than diagnostic tools. Consequently, the professional standards for screening tools are lower than those for diagnostic tools. For example, it may be acceptable for a screening tool to have reliability coefficients in the .80s, whereas you would expect diagnostic tools to have reliability coefficients in the .90s (Salvia et al., 2017). The reason why a lower professional standard exists is that screening tools are often used for low-stake decisions (e.g., additional support), whereas diagnostic tools are often used for high-stake decisions (e.g., special education eligibility). Therefore, examiners should thoroughly read the examiner manual and determine whether the tool should be used for screening purposes. In addition, examiners should evaluate the number of Type I and Type II errors produced by the tool. A Type I error represents a false positive in which the tool inaccurately suggests that an individual has a condition when they really do not. In contrast, a Type II error represents a false negative in which the tool inaccurately suggests that an individual does not have a condition when they really do. For preschool screening purposes, an examiner may favor a higher percentage of Type I errors than Type II errors as the benefits of the additional support may outweigh the potential costs associated with overidentification (Emmons & Alfonso, 2005).

> **DON'T FORGET 3.1**
>
> Screening tools should have reliability coefficients of 0.80 or higher for making low-stake decisions for young children (Salvia et al., 2017).

Due to the ease of use of screening tools, paired with the increase in legislation that has favored early identification and intervention, it is easy to see how they have gained favorable appeal. As a result, the number of preschool screening tools has increased over the past several decades. A few commonly used preschool screening tools are the Developmental Indicators for the Assessment of Learning – Fourth Edition (DIAL-4; Mardell & Goldenberg, 2011), the Clinical Evaluation of Language Fundamentals Preschool – Third Edition Screening Test (CELF Preschool-3 Screening Test; Wiig et al., 2020), and the Bayley Scales of Infant and Toddler Development Screening Test (Bayley-4 Screening Test; Bayley & Aylward, 2019). If these tools, or others, are used appropriately and signify that a young child is "at-risk" of developing further challenges, remedial interventions typically commence. To measure whether an intervention is effective, examiners are encouraged to use progress monitoring tools.

PROGRESS MONITORING

After a young child begins receiving an intervention, it is important to measure whether the intervention is effective. To assist in doing so, examiners are encouraged to use progress monitoring tools. Progress monitoring tools are quick, easy to administer and score, and provide valuable data to assist examiners in making important decisions for young children. For example, progress monitoring assists an examiner in determining whether the intervention should be continued because the young child is showing growth toward their goal(s), whether the intervention should be modified (e.g., longer duration, more frequent, etc.) because the young child is making growth but not enough to reach their goal(s), or whether the intervention should be discontinued because the young child is not making growth toward their goal(s). As a result, examiners can be flexible and nimble in their practices so that they maximize their time working with young children and not wasting time on an intervention that is ineffective.

There are several factors that examiners may want to consider when choosing progress monitoring tools (See Rapid Reference 3.2). First, when selecting a progress monitoring tool, examiners should make sure that it is reflective of the skill or outcome they want to measure. Furthermore, the progress monitoring tool should reflect the skills or outcomes that the intervention is designed to address. For example, if a young child is identified as being "at-risk" for phonemic awareness difficulties, the intervention should specifically address phonemic awareness and the progress monitoring tool should measure phonemic awareness. It is our experiences that the lack of alignment between screening tools, intervention selection, and progress monitoring tools leads to inaccurate decisions about the effectiveness of the intervention.

≡ Rapid Reference 3.2 Progress Monitoring Tools Should Be

- Reflective of the skill and/or outcome you intend to measure
- Sensitive to change
- Administered frequently (e.g., weekly, biweekly)

Second, progress monitoring tools should be sensitive to change. Sensitivity to change refers to the tool's ability to detect subtle changes over a short period of time. If, for example, a progress monitoring tool is not sensitive to change, examiners may mistakenly conclude that an intervention is not effective, when, it is effective. Third, progress monitoring tools should be administered relatively frequently. For example, it is common that progress monitoring tools are administered once a week, or every other week. The increased frequency of administration allows examiners to make on-the-spot decisions regarding whether an intervention should be continued, monitored, or discarded in a timely manner.

If a young child is receiving an intervention and not improving, it may be indicative that the child has a disability. Therefore, examiners should consider completing a comprehensive evaluation to determine the most appropriate way to proceed. A comprehensive evaluation should include multiple sources, multiple methods, and occur across multiple settings and often relies on data from diagnostic tools (Alfonso et al., 2020; Engler et al., 2020).

Diagnostic Tools

One of the common elements of a comprehensive evaluation is the use of diagnostic tools. By diagnostic tools, we are referring to standardized, norm-referenced tests. These tests can be used to evaluate young children to determine whether their performance is consistent with young children of a similar demographic or whether their performance is divergent. If their performance is divergent, it may be indicative of a disability. Therefore, diagnostic tools are used to make high-stake decisions that may have a lasting impact on a young child's future. Given the gravity of these decisions, examiners are encouraged to evaluate critically their diagnostic tools to ensure that they are appropriate for use. To assist in doing so, examiners should evaluate the qualitative and quantitative characteristics of their diagnostic tools while also being mindful of the theoretical make-up, cultural loadings, and linguistic demands of the tool.

Qualitative Characteristics

Chapter 2 (this volume) may have been the first time reading about the importance of evaluating the qualitative characteristics of diagnostic tools. The need to evaluate the qualitative characteristics of diagnostic tools originated just over two decades ago (Alfonso & Flanagan, 1999). In their original work, Alfonso and Flanagan (1999) clearly articulated how strong qualitative characteristics can enhance the testing experience for examiners and examinees alike. Additionally, our experiences working with young children have been that diagnostic tools with strong qualitative characteristics assist examiners in building rapport with examinees. As such, the qualitative characteristics (see Rapid Reference 2.4, this volume) continue to remain as imperative today as they were back then.

There are 10 qualitative characteristics that examiners should be familiar with when assessing young children. Five of the qualitative characteristics focus on test characteristics that are designed to keep a young child's attention throughout the testing session. They include having attractive test materials, having efficient administration procedures, having suitable directions for young children, having opportunities to teach tasks, and having alternative stopping rules. Collectively, these qualitative characteristics are responsive to developmental literature discussing the need to accommodate young children's shorter attention span to maximize interest in educational tasks (Callaghan & Reich, 2020). A list of attention-related qualitative characteristics can be seen in Rapid Reference 3.3 below.

≡ Rapid Reference 3.3 Attention-Related Qualitative Characteristics

- Attractive test materials
- Efficient administration procedures
- Suitable directions for young children
- Opportunities to teach tasks
- Alternative stopping rules

The remaining five qualitative characteristics are related to the language demands placed on young children. Furthermore, two of the five involve limiting the expressive and receptive language requirements of a task unless the task is specifically designed to assess language. For example, a task that only requires a one- or two-word response or allows the young child to point at an answer limits the expressive language requirements of a task. Similarly, directions that are short and simple limit the receptive language requirements of a task. It is also important for a test to have nonverbal scores available unless the test is designed to assess language. The remaining language-related qualitative characteristics include having a test that can be translated or adapted to other languages and having an appropriate degree of cultural loadings and linguistic demands measured within the test. It is imperative for examiners to be cognizant of language-related qualitative characteristics so that the examiner can be sure that tests appropriately measure the constructs that they are designed to measure. A list of language-related qualitative characteristics can be seen in Rapid Reference 3.4 below.

≣ Rapid Reference 3.4 Language-Related Qualitative Characteristics

- Limit expressive language requirements unless assessing language
- Limit receptive language requirements unless assessing language
- Incorporate nonverbal score(s) unless assessing language
- Translation or adaptation available in other languages
- Appropriate degree of language demands and cultural loadings

Quantitative Characteristics

In addition to evaluating the qualitative characteristics of diagnostic tools, it is also imperative to evaluate the quantitative (i.e., psychometric) characteristics. Chapter 2 (this volume) introduced readers to the critical importance of evaluating the psychometric properties of tests and provided evaluative criteria in Table 2.2 to assist examiners in doing so. The following section reinforces and briefly expands upon the evaluative criteria as they are necessary for the responsible assessment of young children. Additionally, the information presented here should complement the discussion from Chapter 2.

In a seminal article within the field of assessment writ-large, Bracken (1988) discussed 10 psychometric reasons why tests purporting to measure the same construct (e.g., cognition, motor, language, etc.) may produce different, or mixed, results. While an in-depth discussion of all 10 reasons is beyond the scope of this chapter due to space limitations, there are several we highlight that have direct relevance to the accuracy of test's results. Further, examiners should be aware of the following psychometric reasons as they can impact assessment results.

The first quantitative characteristic (i.e., reason) involves a test's floor, which Bracken described as the floor effect. In essence, the floor effect describes the bottom echelon of scores that can be obtained on a test. That is, the floor effect involves the corresponding standard/scaled score a young child obtains if they do not answer any test items correctly (or very few items). Evaluating a test's floor is imperative when assessing young children as previous research has shown that test floors at the preschool age range are generally more problematic than other psychometric issues (Flanagan & Alfonso, 1995). If a test does not have a sufficiently low test floor, a young child who answers relatively few test items correctly will have an inflated standard/scaled score. Therefore, to prevent this from occurring test developers should ensure that the test has a sufficient number of easy items so that test performance could be differentiated easily at the lowest level of performance.

> ## CAUTION 3.1
>
> A test with an insufficient floor will result in an inflated test performance.

The second quantitative characteristic involves a test's ceiling, which Bracken described as the ceiling effect. The ceiling effect is similar to the floor effect; however, it corresponds with the highest standard/scaled score a young child obtains if they answer all test items correctly (or mostly all items). Whereas the floor effect is relevant and necessary to evaluate when testing a young child with suspected disabilities, the ceiling effect is relevant and necessary to evaluate when testing a young child with suspected giftedness (Engler & Alfonso, 2020). Consider the following practical example of when an examiner's test choice should reflect an evaluation of the ceiling effect. The examiner is evaluating a young child who is 4 years, 11 months as part of an evaluation for accelerated programming in kindergarten. The examiner has two versions of a test available where one version is normed for young children 3 years–5 years whereas the other version is normed for young children 4 years, 6 months to 7 years. In this example, the examiner should choose the latter, as there are more items at the higher performance level than the former.

> ## DON'T FORGET 3.2
>
> When evaluating a young child for gifted and talented programs, it is necessary that the test has a sufficient ceiling.

The third quantitative characteristic Bracken refers to is called item gradients. Item gradients can be difficult to understand yet are like a test's floor and ceiling. While a test's floor and ceiling are necessary to differentiate performance at the lowest and highest levels of performance, respectively, item gradients refer to a test's ability to differentiate performance within the "typical" range of performance. Moreover, a well-developed test should have a sufficient number of items within each subtest so that subtle raw score changes (e.g., 1-point) do not lead to a large change in standard/scaled scores (Bracken & Theodore, 2020). For example, if a young child obtained a raw score of 12 on a subtest, the corresponding standard/scaled score should not be significantly different than a same-aged child who obtained a raw score of 13. Therefore, a well-developed test adequately covers the range of skills necessary to appropriately assess a domain/construct.

While the first three quantitative characteristics focus on a test's ability to differentiate performance at all ranges of functioning, the next two characteristics focus on the test's normative data. Bracken (1988) described the importance of the layout of a normative table. In particular, Bracken recommended that examiners evaluate whether significant differences in standard/scaled scores would occur if a young child was tested on two consecutive days. For example, most normative tables are divided into age ranges. For the sake of this example, let us assume that a normative table is broken into 6-month age ranges (i.e., 3 years to 3 years, 5 months, 29 days). If a young child 3 years, 5 months, 29 days is tested and obtains a subtest raw score of 12, the corresponding standard/scaled score should not significantly differ if the young child was tested the next day, thus being compared to the 3 years 6 month to 3 years, 11 months, 29 days age range.

In addition to the layout of a normative table, the exactness of the age ranges is important for examiners to consider, especially when testing young children. In particular, research has shown that 1–3-month age ranges are most appropriate, especially when making high-stake decisions for young children (Spector, 1999). The reason why such a small age range is necessary is that young children go through rapid changes in development (Alfonso et al., 2020). For example, those with young children of their own or those who work frequently with young children may have noticed that the child is crawling one day and taking their first steps the next day. Given that young children experience such quick changes in development, having small age ranges improves the accuracy of scores.

Examiners should be cognizant of whether the normative sample accurately represents the population it was based upon. One of the strengths of using a standardized, norm-referenced test is the ability to generalize the test results of an individual to the population (Salvia et al., 2017). If, however, the normative sample does not accurately represent the population, inaccurate results and/or interpretations are likely to occur. Therefore, examiners should critically evaluate the normative sample to ensure that the young children they are testing are represented. Similarly, Bracken (1988) cautioned examiners to evaluate the publication date of a test as tests published at different times may yield different results. This is partially related to the *Flynn Effect* where research has shown that the population's IQ increases over time (Billeiter et al., 2022). Consequently, tests should be renormed periodically (i.e., every 10 years) to account for such increases.

DON'T FORGET 3.3

Normative sample data should be updated approximately every 10 years to avoid the Flynn Effect.

The final quantitative characteristics to be discussed in this chapter are reliability and validity. Reliability refers to the consistency of test scores, whereas validity refers to the degree to which test scores measure the attributes they purport to measure. The reliability of a test can be evidenced in several ways which involve consistency across items, over time, and across examiners. First, to measure the reliability of a test across items, internal consistency is used. Internal consistency is often calculated using Cronbach's alpha (Sattler, 2008). Second, to measure the reliability of a test over time, test–retest reliability is often used. Test–retest reliability involves administering a test at one point in time, and then again at a second point in time. The scores are then correlated resulting in a coefficient. Third, to measure the reliability of a test across examiners, interrater reliability is used. Interrater reliability involves multiple raters scoring test items and is the degree to which the multiple raters agree.

Similar to reliability, the validity of a test can be evidenced in several ways. Validity refers to the degree to which a test accurately measures what it states that it measures. A test, however, should not be thought of as either valid or not valid. Rather, there are evidences that can support a test's use. Fortunately, the *Standards for Educational and Psychological Testing* (American Educational Research Association et al., 2014) provides guidance for examiners regarding different sources of validity to reference. AERA et al. (2014) provided several evidences for validity that examiners should evaluate prior to administering a test. The first evidence of validity is content-oriented evidence. Content-oriented evidence involves the creation of the content of a test. As an example, a test publisher may describe the procedures for developing test content (e.g., expert panels, expert reviewers, literature review, etc.) to support that the test is measuring the domain/construct it was designed to measure. The second evidence of validity is regarding cognitive processes. For example, if a test is designed to measure a specific set of abilities, a test publisher may have researchers interview test takers and ask questions regarding how that individual approached each task. Additionally, the test publisher may have individuals evaluate test taker responses to see if the responses are consistent with the expected task.

The third evidence for validity is regarding the internal structure of the test (AERA et al., 2014). For example, if a test purports to measure cognitive abilities, evidence regarding the internal structure of the test may show an exploratory and/or confirmatory factor analysis that demonstrates consistency with an underlying cognitive theory (e.g., Cattell-Horn-Carroll Theory). If, however, the test is unidimensional, the test publishers may support this with a single-factor model. The fourth evidence for validity is regarding relationships with conceptually related constructs. Therefore, a test publisher may provide evidence for their test by showing that the test is highly correlated with other published tests measuring similar constructs. For example, a newly created test that is designed to measure motor abilities (i.e., fine motor and gross motor) should be highly correlated with a well-established and supported test of motor abilities.

The fifth evidence for validity is regarding relationships with other criteria (AERA et al., 2014). An example that is commonly used by test publishers is the prediction of some type of outcome related to the results of a test. For example, if a test publisher created a test of cognitive abilities, a source of evidence regarding relationships with other criteria may be the relationship between the test's overall score and membership within a gifted and talented program 3 years later. The sixth and final evidence for validity is regarding the consequences of tests. All tests have intended consequence and unintended consequences. It is incumbent that tests published provide evidence for their claims regarding both.

Summary of Quantitative Characteristics

There are many quantitative considerations examiners should evaluate prior to administering diagnostic tools. They include a test's floor, ceiling, item gradients, the standardization sample (including normative table layouts), evidence for reliability, and evidence for validity. The previous section included a description regarding what each quantitative consideration is, why it is important, and how it may influence the test's results. What was missing, however, was a systematic way to evaluate the quantitative characteristics of a test. Fortunately, researchers have worked diligently to develop such criteria. While an in-depth discussion regarding the creation of the criteria is precluded from this chapter due to space considerations, we would like to draw the reader's attention to Table 2.2 (this volume) as a reference. Readers are encouraged to use these criteria to evaluate the overall quality of a test. Readers should be cognizant that no test is perfect, and we have not come across a test that exceeds all expectations. Rather, the cumulative evaluation of a test may help examiners decipher which test to use and why.

CAUTION 3.2

A standardized, norm-referenced test should not be considered valid or not valid.

Theoretical Characteristics

The understanding of cognitive theory has been rapidly advancing over the past couple of decades (see, e.g., McGrew et al., 2023; Naglieri & Otero, 2018; Schneider & McGrew, 2018; Sternberg, 2018). That said, perhaps the most sophisticated and validated cognitive theory is the Cattell-Horn-Carroll Theory of Cognitive Abilities (CHC Theory). In basic terms, the CHC Theory is a three-stratum hierarchical model. The bottom level of the hierarchy is called stratum one and represents narrow abilities. Narrow abilities are task-related measures, which are often observed within individual subtests. The middle level of the hierarchy is called stratum two and represents broad abilities. Broad abilities are a related cluster of narrow abilities and are often synonymous with composite/cluster scores. The top of the hierarchy is called stratum three and represents g or general cognitive ability. g is synonymous with a full-scale cognitive score (i.e., full-scale intelligence quotient, general intellectual ability, etc.). Interested readers are encouraged to see Schneider and McGrew (2018) for the most current iteration of CHC Theory.

While CHC Theory has been advancing and evolving, so too has its role in the development of cognitive tests. In fact, even tests that were once atheoretical in nature (i.e., Wechsler Scales) are now including CHC Theory in their interpretive framework. Although the application of CHC Theory in test development has traditionally focused on school-aged children and been extrapolated downward in its application to preschool-aged children (Ford et al., 2012), there is growing evidence to support the use of CHC Theory with preschool-age children (Tusing, & Ford, 2004).

Recently, Engler and Alfonso (2020) reviewed the theoretical underpinnings of five commonly used cognitive tests for preschool-aged children. The review identified the number of CHC Theory broad and narrow abilities that are measured within each test. The review indicated that preschool-aged cognitive tests varied considerably in the number of broad and narrow abilities measured. Therefore, examiners should be cautioned that not all cognitive tests measure the same abilities. As a result, we recommend that examiners review the theoretical underpinnings of tests (particularly when assessing cognitive abilities) and utilize the test that most comprehensively addresses the referral question.

> **DON'T FORGET 3.4**
>
> Not all preschool-aged cognitive tests measure the same theoretical constructs.

Cultural and Linguistic Characteristics

Contrary to popular belief, early childhood development is not dependent on the racial and/or ethnical make-up of a child (Ortiz & Wong, 2020). Moreover, regardless of race and ethnicity, one can expect young children from various states, countries, and continents to develop cognitive, language, motor, adaptive, and behavior/emotional skills along a similar developmental trajectory. As such, the way in which examiners evaluate young children should be culturally responsive and may differ based on several important considerations. One of the most important considerations for examiners to consider is the degree to which cultural loading and linguistic demands impact test performance.

Cultural Loadings and Linguistic Demands

One important consideration when assessing a young child who is culturally and linguistically diverse is to evaluate the degree of cultural and linguistic loadings for each subtest within a test. Furthermore, if a test and/or subtest(s) is/are shown to measure a high degree of culture and/or language, the results of the test may be erroneous as they may not be purely measuring the construct that the test purports to measure (e.g., visual-spatial processing, working memory, etc.). Engler and Alfonso (2020) provided a systematic way to do so when they comprehensively reviewed five preschool cognitive tests. As part of the comprehensive evaluation, Engler and Alfonso used the Cultural-Language Interpretive Matrix of the Cross-Battery Assessment System Software (X-BASS; Flanagan et al., 2017) to determine the cultural loadings and linguistic demands for each subtest within the five cognitive tests. The authors then categorized each subtest as a combination of either high, moderate, or low cultural loadings and either high, moderate, or low linguistic demands. While there is not an exact science (e.g., cut-point) for the number of subtests that should have low cultural loadings and low linguistic demands, examiners can use this information in context to make decisions about the appropriateness of a test. For example, results of the evaluation showed that some preschool cognitive tests may be more appropriate than others when evaluating young children who are culturally and linguistically diverse. While this review focused on cognitive tests, the same procedure can be used when evaluating the cultural loadings and linguistic demands of other tests (e.g., neuropsychological tests).

SUMMARY

The responsible assessment of young children is not easy. It requires a nuanced approach and understanding of assessment practices paired with a thorough understanding of early childhood development. As evidenced throughout this chapter, there are several considerations for examiners to pay careful attention to throughout the assessment process. For example, examiners should know that there are various purposes associated with assessment, including screening, progress monitoring, and diagnosis/eligibility decision-making. Each of the purposes has unique considerations due to their function and desired outcomes. Additionally, each has strengths and weaknesses associated with its use. Therefore, examiners should be familiar with the strengths and weaknesses so that they may use them appropriately.

The bulk of the chapter emphasized several important considerations when evaluating diagnostic tools (i.e., standardized, norm-referenced tests) as they are often used for high-stake decision-making. There are several factors that must be considered when evaluating the quality of a diagnostic test. First, a high-quality test for young children should be designed with young children in mind. While this may seem intuitive, tests for young children were often originally designed for school-aged children and then extrapolated to preschool-aged children. Furthermore, it should be interactive, varied, and capable of holding a young child's attention. Second, a high-quality test should have a number of quantitative characteristics that support its use. For example, it should be recently published, be able to differentiate performance across abilities, and be adequately reliable and valid. Third, a high-quality test should be theoretically driven (when applicable) and measure theoretical constructs with sufficient depth and breadth needed to guide interpretation and inform the decision-making process. Fourth, a high-quality test should take into account the cultural loading and linguistic demands of the test. This ensures that the test is measuring what it is designed to measure and that non-native English-speaking children are not disadvantaged.

It should be noted that a test incorporating everything within this chapter does not currently exist. Furthermore, each test clearly has its own strengths and weaknesses. Therefore, examiners must also understand that not all tests are created equal, and some tests clearly outperform others. Consequently, examiners should use information gained from this chapter, paired with their own professional knowledge and experience, to evaluate the overall quality of the test. In particular, examiners should guide their decision-making process with a specific referral question or questions in mind and a thorough understanding of the young child in mind. From there, the examiner can use that context to evaluate whether a test will appropriately and accurately answer the referral question(s).

🖋 TEST YOURSELF 🖋

1. **Which of the following laws requires a free and appropriate public education for individuals with disabilities:**
   (a) Head Start/Early Head Start
   (b) Every Student Succeeds Act
   (c) Education for All Handicapped Children Act
   (d) None of the above

2. **Screening tools are less expensive than diagnostic tools.**
   (a) True
   (b) False

3. **Progress monitoring tools should be:**
   (a) Reflective of the skills you intended to measure
   (b) Sensitive to change
   (c) Administered frequently
   (d) All of the above

4. **Evaluating the qualitative characteristics of tests is less important than evaluating the quantitative characteristics of tests.**
   (a) True
   (b) False

5. **Which of the following is a qualitative characteristic of a test:**
   (a) Reliability
   (b) Opportunities to teach tasks
   (c) Test ceiling
   (d) Item gradients

6. **Test floors are used to differentiate performance at the lower levels of functioning.**
   (a) True
   (b) False

7. **An inadequate test ceiling deflates performance at the higher levels of functioning.**
   (a) True
   (b) False

8. **A test should be renormed approximately every:**
   (a) Year
   (b) 3 years
   (c) 5 years
   (d) 10 years

9. **CHC Theory is a three-stratum hierarchical model.**
   (a) True
   (b) False

10. **Cultural loadings and linguistic demands should not be considered when evaluating a test.**
    (a) True
    (b) False

Answers: 1. c; 2. a; 3. d; 4. b; 5. b; 6. a; 7. a; 8. d; 9. a; 10. b

REFERENCES

Alfonso, V. C., Engler, J. R., & Lepore, J. C. (2020). Assessing and evaluating young children: Developmental domains and methods. In V. C. Alfonso & G. J. DuPaul (Eds.), *Healthy development in young children: Evidence-based interventions for early education* (pp. 13–44). American Psychological Association.

Alfonso, V. C., Engler, J. R., & Turner, A. D. (2022). *Essential of Bayley-4 assessment*. Wiley Publishing.

Alfonso, V. C., & Flanagan, D. P. (1999). Assessment of cognitive functioning in preschoolers. In E. V. Nuttall, I. Romero, & J. Kalesnik (Eds.), *Assessing and screening preschoolers* (2nd ed., pp. 186–217). Allyn & Bacon.

American Educational Research Association, American Psychological Association, & National Council on Measurement in Education. (2014). *Standards for educational and psychological testing*. American Educational Research Association.

Bayley, N., & Aylward, G. P. (2019). *Bayley scales of infant and toddler development screening test*. Pearson.

Billeiter, K. B., Froiland, J. M., Allen, J. P., & Hajovsky, D. B. (2022). Neurodiversity and intelligence: Evaluating the Flynn effect in children with autism spectrum disorder. *Child Psychiatry and Human Development, 53*, 919–927. https://doi.org/10.1007/s10578-021-01175-w

Bracken, B. A. (1988). Ten psychometric reasons why similar tests produce dissimilar results. *Journal of School Psychology, 26*, 155–166.

Bracken, B. A., & Theodore, L. A. (2020). Creating the optimal preschool testing situation. In V. C. Alfonso, B. A. Bracken, & R. J. Nagle (Eds.), *Psychoeducational assessment of preschool children* (5th ed., pp. 55–75). Routledge.

Callaghan, M. N., & Reich, S. M. (2020). Applying a developmental lens to educational game designs for preschoolers. *International Journal of Mobile and Blended Learning, 12*(2), 1–15.

Emmons, M., & Alfonso, V. C. (2005). A critical review of the technical characteristics of current preschool screening batteries. *Journal of Psychoeducational Assessment, 23*, 111–127.

Engler, J. R., & Alfonso, V. C. (2020). Cognitive assessment of preschool children: A pragmatic review of theoretical, quantitative, and qualitative characteristics. In V. C. Alfonso, B. A. Bracken, & R. J. Nagle (Eds.), *Psychoeducational assessment of preschool children* (5th ed., pp. 226–249). Routledge.

Engler, J. R., Alfonso, V. C., White, J. M., & Ray, C. D. (2020). Assessing social-emotional abilities of preschool-aged children within a social-emotional framework. *Perspectives on Early Childhood Psychology and Education, 5*(1), 171–197.

Flanagan, D. P., & Alfonso, V. C. (1995). A critical review of the technical characteristics of new and recently revised intelligence tests for preschool children. *Journal of Psychoeducational Assessment, 13*, 66–90.

Flanagan, D. P., Ortiz, S. O., & Alfonso, V. C. (2017). *Cross-battery assessment software system (X-BASS)*. (Version 2.0). [Computer Software]. John Wiley and Sons.

Ford, L., Kozey, M. L., & Negreiros, J. (2012). Cognitive assessment in early childhood: Theoretical and practice perspectives. In D. P. Flanagan & P. L. Harrison (Eds.), *Contemporary intellectual assessment: Theories, tests, and issues* (3rd ed., pp. 585–622). The Guilford Press.

Mardell, C., & Goldenberg, D. S. (2011). *Developmental indicators for the assessment of learning* (4th ed.). Pearson.

McGrew, K. S., Schneider, W. J., Decker, S. L., & Bulut, O. (2023). A psychometric network analysis of CHC intelligence measures: Implications for research, theory, and interpretation of broad CHC scores 'beyond g'. *Journal of Intelligence, 11*(1), 1–33. https://doi.org/10.3390/jintelligence11010019

Merriam-Webster. (n.d.). Responsible. Retrieved March 13, 2023 from https://www.merriam-webster.com/dictionary/responsible.

Naglieri, J. A., & Otero, T. M. (2018). Redefining intelligence with the planning, attention, simultaneous, and successive theory of neurocognitive processes. In D. P. Flanagan & E. M. McDonough (Eds.), *Contemporary intellectual assessment: Theories, tests, and issues* (4th ed., pp. 195–218). The Guilford Press.

Office of Elementary & Secondary Education. (2023). Preschool development grant – birth through five. Retrieved June 26, 2023, from https://oese.ed.gov/offices/office-of-discretionary-grants-support-services/innovation-early-learning/preschool-development-grants/.

Office of Head Start. (2023). Head start services. Retrieved June 26, 2023,from https://www.acf.hhs.gov/ohs/about/head-start.

Ortiz, S. O., & Wong, J. Y. T. (2020). Psychoeducational assessment of culturally and linguistically diverse preschool children. In V. C. Alfonso, B. A. Bracken, & R. J. Nagle (Eds.), *Psychoeducational assessment of preschool children* (5th ed., pp. 346–374). Routledge.

Salvia, J., Ysseldyke, J. E., & Witmer, S. (2017). *Assessment in special and inclusive education* (13th ed.). Cengage.

Sattler, J. (2008). *Assessment of children: Cognitive foundations* (5th ed.). Author.

Schmitt, A., Wodrich, D. L., & Lorenzi-Quigley, L. (2020). Current status of pediatric topics in five school psychology journals: Publication trends between 2002 and 2019. *School Psychology, 35*(3), 171–178. https://doi.org/10.1037/spq0000346

Schneider, W. J., & McGrew, K. S. (2018). The Cattell-Horn-Carroll theory of cognitive abilities. In D. P. Flanagan & E. M. McDonough (Eds.), *Contemporary intellectual assessment: Theories, tests, and issues* (4th ed., pp. 73–163). The Guilford Press.

Spector, J. E. (1999). Precision of age norms in tests used to assess preschool children. *Psychology in the Schools, 36,* 459–471.

Sternberg, R. J. (2018). The triarchic theory of successful intelligence. In D. P. Flanagan & E. M. McDonough (Eds.), *Contemporary intellectual assessment: Theories, tests, and issues* (4th ed., pp. 174–194). The Guilford Press.

Tusing, M. E., & Ford, L. (2004). Examining preschool cognitive abilities using a CHC framework. *International Journal of Testing, 4*(2), 91–114.

Wiig, E. H., Secord, W. A., & Semel, E. (2020). *Clinical evaluation of language fundamentals preschool-3 screening test.* Pearson.

Four

ASSESSMENT OF IDEA DEVELOPMENTAL DOMAINS

Federal law has had a significant impact on the assessment of young children and the available measurement tools. As described in other chapters of this volume, the Individuals with Disability Education Improvement Act of 2004 (IDEA) and its predecessors outlined the eligibility standards for intervention services for young children. Young children must be found eligible for services through evaluation, most often occurring within a comprehensive assessment of all developmental domains as described by federal and state laws. The five developmental domains included under IDEA are physical development, cognitive development, communication development, social and/or emotional development, and adaptive development (IDEA, 2004 Section 300.8 (b)). Assessment tools used with young children, therefore, typically align with these developmental domains.

When a young child evidences a delay in one or more developmental domains, examiners must determine the degree of delay, whether it is isolated to one domain, or is more global in nature. Therefore, comprehensive assessments of young children should include all developmental domains. As described in Chapter 2 of this volume,

> ### DON'T FORGET 4.1
>
> The five IDEA developmental domains include physical development, cognitive development, communication development, social and/or emotional development, and adaptive development.

Essentials of Assessing Infants, Toddlers, and Preschoolers, First Edition.
Brittany A. Dale, Joseph R. Engler, and Vincent C. Alfonso.
© 2025 John Wiley & Sons, Inc. Published 2025 by John Wiley & Sons, Inc.

comprehensive assessments can include direct measurement of a child's skills, parent report of behaviors, and direct observation of what the young child can do during an evaluation. Under IDEA, comprehensive assessments can occur during early childhood (i.e., birth to 2 years) or during preschool (i.e., ages 3 through 5 years and transition to kindergarten).

Not only does assessment assist in determining eligibility for early intervention or special education preschool services, but it also helps a family understand if their child is ready for kindergarten. School readiness is considered a multifaceted construct that includes language and literacy development, mathematical knowledge, physical development, and social–emotional skills (Ferretti & Bub, 2017; Hojnoski & Missall, 2020). Once a child enters preschool, foundational pre-academic skills are assessed informally by school staff, while formal assessment tools are available for examiners.

This chapter provides an overview of the assessment of young children across the various IDEA developmental domains (i.e., physical, cognitive, communication, social–emotional, and adaptive). First, an overview of each of the five IDEA developmental domains is presented with a brief description of a few common tests used during the assessment and evaluation of a young child. Then, we review comprehensive developmental tests used during an assessment for developmental delays and help assist in special education and early intervention eligibility determination. Lastly, we discuss the importance of assessing functional pre-academics in this population and provide a summary of some common tools to assess these skills. A comprehensive review of each developmental domain is beyond the scope of this chapter and the purpose of this volume; however, we provide a comprehensive measure of tests that can be used to assess the IDEA developmental domains in the Appendix.

DOMAIN SPECIFIC ASSESSMENT

As described above, direct measurement of the developmental domains is imperative during an assessment for educational eligibility and to help inform intervention plans in early intervention and preschool settings. Assessment tools may include individually administered tests, interview forms, rating scales, and observational methods. The type of test utilized will depend on the developmental domain being assessed. The following sections provide a summary of the developmental skills of a young child by domain as well as some of the instruments used when assessing that domain.

Physical Development

Physical development includes motor skills, sensory processing, and feeding. This section focuses on motor skill development and the corresponding tests utilized during the assessment of a young child. Sensory processing evaluation is briefly discussed. For information on pediatric feeding disorders and the corresponding evaluations used to determine diagnosis and intervention, see Goday et al., 2019, Kovacic et al., 2020, and the Feeding Matters Organization (https://www.feedingmatters.org/; Feeding Matters, 2024).

Motor skill development (i.e., fundamental motor skills) follows a typical pattern in children. Young children initially develop the base skills (e.g., adjust their bodies, develop strength, refine their posture, etc.) that will contribute to all later motor movement. Motor skills are typically divided into gross and fine motor skills. These skills include moving the body through space by running and jumping, manipulating objects such as balls with the hands and feet, and grasping (Goodway et al., 2010). See Rapid Reference 4.1 for definitions and examples of fine and gross motor skills in young children.

Rapid Reference 4.1 Motor Skills Assessed During a Developmental Evaluation

Skill	Definition	Examples
Gross Motor	Movements in which large body muscles are used	Sitting, walking and running, standing, creeping, and crawling
Fine Motor	Movements in which small muscles are used	Grasping, receiving, and dropping objects
Perceptual Motor	Recognizing the stimulus and interpretating what it means followed by movement. It is also coordination and sequences of movement to achieve a goal.	Writing, dexterity, balance, and strength
Visual Motor	The ability to use vision to perform motor tasks	Hand-eye coordination used to copy designs and handwriting

Note: From Veiskarami et al., 2021; D'Costa & Hanig, 2014; Coallier et al., 2014; Santos et al., 2020; Taverna et al., 2021

Infants progress through stages to learn to adjust their bodies in relation to gravity, develop strength to refine their posture, and ultimately learn to move themselves through space. Fine motor skills coordinate with gross motor skills for young children to learn to pick up objects and manipulate them appropriately. Sex differences in motor skill development begin at an early age and are consistent through the early childhood years (Kokstejn et al., 2017). For example, preschool-aged girls outperform boys on tasks of grasping and visual-motor integration (Dourou et al., 2017), whereas boys have significantly better object control skills (Goodway et al., 2010).

Assessment of fine and gross motor skill development commonly occurs for infants, toddlers, and preschoolers with developmental delays. Occupational therapists (OTs) are the experts in fine motor and sensory motor skills, along with activities of daily living, whereas physical therapists (PTs) specialize in gross motor skills. Within the preschool setting, the initial concern and corresponding referral question ultimately drives which related service providers become involved in the assessment process. For instance, not all children with developmental delays exhibit a deficit in gross motor skills; therefore, a PT is not always a member of the assessment team. Additionally, school psychologists are often trained in the assessment of visual-motor integration skills and are competent in the assessment of various fine motor skills. As such, OTs may not be needed on all assessment teams.

> **DON'T FORGET 4.2**
>
> In a multidisciplinary setting, occupational therapists assess a young child's fine motor skills, and physical therapists assess their gross motor skills.

The importance of motor skills in early childhood is undebatable. Early childhood educators consider fine motor skills a necessary component of school readiness, and accurate assessment of fine motor skills is vital to implementing early motor skills interventions (Cameron et al., 2012). Fine motor skills have been associated with cognitive abilities, language skills, and social–emotional difficulties, and delays in fine motor skills predict referral to special education (Cameron et al., 2012). Children who perform better on fine motor assessments in preschool also perform better on kindergarten readiness assessments, and motor skills in kindergarten predict later reading and math achievement in young children (Carlson et al., 2013). Children utilize visual-motor skills to complete functional tasks such as self-care skills and schoolwork. Research suggests an association between academic achievement and visual-motor integration skills; fine motor skills, without the visual-integration component, are less associated with academic achievement (Carlson et al., 2013).

Motor assessment is also an integral component during the assessment of children with specific neurodevelopmental disorders or medical conditions (discussed more in Chapter 5 of this volume) and can assist in eligibility placement and intervention planning. For instance, infants and toddlers with motor skill delays are more likely to have global developmental delays compared to those with autism spectrum disorder or general language delays (Dale et al., 2022). For premature children, motor delays persist from preschool into early elementary school, which has implications for school-based intervention services.

Fine Motor Skills

During a fine motor skills assessment, OTs evaluate the fine, visual, and perceptual motor skill development of a child. As summarized in Rapid Reference 4.1 earlier, fine motor skills involve the small muscles and include how children recognize a stimulus, interpret it, and coordinate movement to achieve a goal (Santos et al., 2020; Veiskarami et al., 2021). During this assessment, OTs often evaluate if a child has developed a dominant hand preference. Most children develop preferred hand dominance between the ages of two and three years; however, approximately 50% of children show signs of hand dominance earlier. Research suggests that children who display a hand preference earlier exhibit advanced developmental cognitive skills (Michel et al., 2016).

Gross Motor Skills

During a gross motor skill assessment, PTs look for deficits in the skills produced by the large muscles of the body. Within the school environment, they assess whether delays in such skills impact a young child's ability to access his or her school environment. This may include walking up and down stairs, moving about the playground safely, and navigating the hallways of a school building. Individual tests of gross motor skills often include domains that assess locomotion and object manipulation/control. Locomotion includes running, skipping, hopping, jumping forward, etc. and object manipulation/control typically refers to ball skills (throw overhand, kick, catch, etc.; Hardy et al., 2010; Salami et al., 2022).

Many tests of motor development include fine and gross motor skills. The following sections describe several common measures utilized by PTs and OTs during a developmental evaluation of a young child. These measures can inform a multidisciplinary team of the physical skills of the young child when determining eligibility for early intervention services, preschool special education services, and other supplemental interventions.

Peabody Developmental Motor Scales, Second Edition (PDMS-2). The Peabody Developmental Motor Scales, Second Edition (PDMS-2; Folio & Fewell, 2000) can be used to assess the fine and gross motor skills of children from birth to age 5:11. Originally published in 1983, the PDMS-2 takes approximately 45–60 minutes to complete. Full administration of the PDMS-2 yields two composite scores, the Fine Motor Quotient and the Gross Motor Quotient, with one overall composite, the Total Motor Quotient. Fine motor skills are assessed through two subtests including the visio-motor integration and grasping subtests. Gross motor skills are broken into four subtests: assessing reflexes, locomotion, object manipulation, and stationary skills. Research suggests the PDMS-2 is superior to motor tests on comprehensive developmental measures when identifying fine motor delay in toddlers under 36 months of age (Lin et al., 2020). Additionally, independent research has verified the reliability and validity of the PDMS-2 with various groups of young children (Lin et al., 2020; van Hartingsveldt et al., 2015).

Beery-Buktenica Developmental Test of Visual-Motor Integration, Sixth Edition (Beery VMI). The Beery-Buktenica Developmental Test of Visual-Motor Integration (Beery VMI), now in its sixth edition (Beery & Beery, 2010), helps assess how individuals integrate their visual and motor skills. Originally published in 1964, the Beery VMI boasts a long history of research support and has been standardized with over 13,000 children and 1,000 adults. The most recent standardization process focused on the assessment of visual-motor integration skills in early childhood (Beery & Beery, 2010). During administration, participants are asked to copy drawings of geometric forms. The scores consist of visual-motor integration, visual perception, and motor coordination. The Beery VMI overall score has been found to be predictive of handwriting speed in preschool children (van Hartinsveldt et al., 2015).

Test of Gross Motor Development, Third Edition (TGMD-3). The Test of Gross Motor Development (TGMD; Ulrich, 1985, 2000, 2019) is one of the most widely used and researched tools for gross motor functioning (Field et al., 2020). Originally published in 1985, the TGMD assesses fundamental motor skills in children 3–10 years old. Now in the third edition, the TGMD-3 (Ulrich, 2019) assesses gross motor skills in the categories of locomotion and ball skills. The Locomotion subtest measures a child's skills at moving his or her body in a coordinated manner, and the Ball Skills subtest measures throwing, striking, and catching movements. The examiner, typically a PT, demonstrates each item, allows the child to practice the item, and then scores the child on critical elements during two scored practice trials. The Locomotion and Ball Skills subtests are combined to create the Gross Motor Composite. Results reveal whether a child has mastered the target skills, which can be useful for intervention planning, progress monitoring, and program evaluation (Field et al., 2020).

Sensory Processing

Sensory experiences are another area often assessed during a multidisciplinary developmental evaluation, typically by the OT. Sensory processing assessments provide early interventionists with knowledge of how a young child experiences their environment through their senses. Young children use body-centered (tactile, proprioceptive, and vestibular), auditory, and visual systems to engage in everyday activities such as playing, eating, and learning (Ayres, 2005). Ayers Sensory Integration Theory identifies how the processing of sensory information impacts a child's adaptive and behavioral functioning (Brown et al., 2023). Dunn's model of sensory processing (1997) is another common framework to understand sensory processing differences in young children. Dunn's model includes variable neurological thresholds for sensory input and either active or passive self-regulation strategies or behavioral responses to the sensory input. As discussed later, these theories provide the foundation for several sensory processing measures.

Appropriate sensory processing skills are essential for social engagement, emotional regulation, adaptive functioning (Brown et al., 2023), and behavior regulation (Brown et al., 2021); therefore, deficits in sensory processing can lead to daily impairment in young children. For instance, sensory processing patterns and deficits can be seen in infants, toddlers, and young children who have a variety of disabilities, including autism, attention deficit hyperactivity disorder, developmental disabilities (Dunn, 2007), and learning disabilities (Estaki et al., 2021). Licciardi and Brown (2023) argue that understanding sensory processing is essential for OTs to build effective intervention programs for young children and their families. The sections below provide a brief overview of two common rating scales used to assess sensory processing in young children. For a comprehensive review of sensory processing measures that can be used with infants and toddlers, see Eeles and colleagues (2013), and for preschoolers, see Jorquera-Cabrera et al. (2017).

DON'T FORGET 4.3

Sensory processing is an important component of a developmental evaluation, which is often assessed by an OT.

Sensory Profile 2. The Sensory Profile 2 (Dunn, 2014) assesses sensory processing in children birth through 14 years, 11 months old. It is the revised version of the original Sensory Profile family of tools (Dunn, 1999), which was considered the most widely used test of sensory processing across disorders (Saulnier & Ventola, 2012). The Sensory Profile included four separate forms to assess the sensory processing of infants, toddlers, children, and adolescents across the home and school environments. Updated to include five forms, the Sensory Profile 2 has separate parent/caregiver report forms for infants, toddlers, and preschoolers: Infant Sensory Profile 2, Toddler Sensory Profile 2, and Child Sensory Profile 2. A Short Sensory Profile 2 and School Companion Sensory Profile 2 are also available, with the latter being appropriate for teachers to complete. Licciardi and Brown (2023) describe the Sensory Profile 2 as a psychometrically sound measure to assess a young child's sensory patterns for the purposes of intervention development, advocacy, and research. They caution that sensory rating scales should be used in conjunction with parent, caregiver, and teacher interviews, as well as behavioral observations of the child to gain a full picture of the young child's sensory processing needs.

Sensory Processing Measure, Second Edition (SPM-2). The Sensory Processing Measure, Second Edition (SPM-2; Parham et al., 2021) is another popular measure used to assess sensory processing in young children. Grounded in Ayers Sensory Integration Theory, the goal of the SPM-2 is to gain a complete picture of an individual's sensory functioning at home, at school, and in the community. There are forms specifically for infants and toddlers from 4-9 months and 10-30 months, and preschool children 2–5 years old. For preschool children, separate forms for home and school are available. Additional forms are available to assess older children and adults up to 87 years old. The SPM-2 provides standard t-scores across six sensory systems, and includes sensory total, planning, and social participation scores. The sensory systems measured are visual, auditory, tactile, olfactory, and gustatory (grouped together), proprioceptive (body awareness), and vestibular (balance and motion) sensory systems. The higher the standard t-score, the greater the difficulty the child has processing the sensory information, ranging from *typical* to *severe difficulties*.

Cognitive Abilities

Cognitive assessment of young children varies depending on the age of the child. Specifically, infant and toddler cognitive abilities are most commonly assessed through the cognitive scale of comprehensive developmental tests. Preschool cognitive abilities (i.e., children ages 2 years, 6 months through 5 years) are typically assessed through traditional cognitive ability measures based on modern intelligence theory (i.e., Cattell-Horn-Carroll Theory [CHC]; Engler & Alfonso, 2020). The following sections discuss the cognitive abilities of young children based on developmental ages.

Infants and Toddlers

Infant and toddler cognitive milestones include attending to and processing information, remembering, and reasoning with and knowing information. These skills are often assessed through the cognitive domain or subtest of a comprehensive developmental test, several of which will be described later in this chapter. At young ages, tests of cognitive abilities assess whether a child attends to stimuli in their environment, reaches toward items, explores items through mouthing and touch, stacks items, searches for hidden items, pretends with toys, and begins to use writing utensils (CDC, 2021). Infant and toddler cognitive ability can be influenced by factors such as infant sleep disturbance (Camerota et al., 2020), motor skills (Michel et al., 2016), prematurity (Kerr-Wilson et al., 2012), birth weight (Alyward, 2002), and access to play materials at home (Miquelote et al., 2012). Enriching activities between parent and infant are positively associated with infant cognitive functioning (Hendry et al., 2022). Furthermore, infant and toddler cognitive abilities are predictive of preschool IQ. Klein-Radukic and Zmyj (2023) found that cognitive scores on the Bayley Scales of Infant and Toddler Development, Third Edition (Bayley, 2006) across the infant and toddler period (6, 9, 18, and 20 months old) predicted IQ on the Wechsler Preschool and Primary Scale of Intelligence, Third Edition (Wechsler, 2002) at 4 years, 2 months old.

Preschoolers

Current tests of preschool cognitive abilities most commonly align with the CHC model of intelligence. CHC theory is a multidimensional, hierarchical model consisting of a general cognitive ability (*g*), broad abilities, and narrow abilities. Narrow abilities are considered specific abilities that cluster together as highly correlated skills to make up the broad abilities. Over 90 narrow abilities have been identified, falling into approximately 17 broad ability categories (Schneider & McGrew, 2018). A more thorough discussion of the CHC model of intelligence is provided in Chapter 4 of this volume.

In a recent review, Engler and Alfonso (2020) summarize the important considerations examiners should make when selecting preschool cognitive tests. These include the cultural and language loading of the test, suitable directions for preschoolers, attractiveness of test materials, learning opportunities to "teach task," efficient administration procedures, inclusion of a nonverbal scale, and alternative stopping rules. In addition to these characteristics, examiners must consider a young child's motor skills when selecting tests of intelligence and interpret findings in relation to those skills (Sotelo-Dynega & Dixon, 2014). For instance, subtests from several common cognitive ability tests include manipulatives such as blocks, puzzle pieces, and cards, and children with fine motor delays may have difficulty holding and maneuvering the manipulatives. Furthermore, Engler and Alfonso also rate the psychometric properties of several common preschool cognitive ability tests, and the reader is encouraged to consult these ratings prior to developing their assessment plan.

> ## CAUTION 4.1
>
> Examiners should not administer cognitive tests that require the use of manipulatives when a young child has motor impairments.

Wechsler Preschool and Primary Scale of Intelligence, Fourth Edition (WPPSI-IV). The Wechsler Preschool and Primary Scale of Intelligence, Fourth Edition (WPPSI-IV; Wechsler, 2012) is an individually administered test of intelligence designed to assess young children ages 2 years, 6 months through 7 years, 7 months. The WPPSI-IV was updated to include cognitive constructs that constitute general intellectual functioning and underlying academic skills development (Wahlstrom et al., 2018) and to align more closely with the CHC theory of intelligence. The WPPSI-IV includes a dynamic conceptualization of intelligence, which recognizes the role of varying abilities. For instance, working memory and processing speed have increasingly been acknowledged as important precursors to higher-order cognitive abilities as well as academic skills (Wahlstrom et al., 2018). The WPPSI was originally published in 1967, and the most recent revision reflects 60% new subtests from its original form. Test stimuli are visually engaging, time to administer was reduced, and tasks to align with more areas of the CHC model (processing speed and working memory) were added. The WPPSI-IV provides examiners the ability to assess comprehensive cognitive abilities in preschool children.

The WPPSI-IV is divided into two age bands with separate protocols. The first age band includes ages 2 years, 6 months through 3 years, 11 months. Young children in this age band can be administered five core subtests and two supplemental subtests. The second age band includes ages 4 years, 0 months through 7 years, 7 months. Children in this age band can be administered up to 15 subtests. The WPPSI-IV yields a Full Scale IQ (FSIQ), Verbal Comprehension Index (VCI), Visual Spatial Index (VSI), and Working Memory Index (WMI) for the 2 year 6 month through 3 years 11 months age band, with an FSIQ, VCI, VSI, WMI, Processing Speed Index (PSI), and Fluid Reasoning Index (FRI) for the older age band.

Woodcock-Johnson-IV Tests of Early Cognitive and Academic Development (ECAD). The Woodcock–Johnson series of assessments added the Tests of Early Cognitive and Academic Development (ECAD; Schrank et al., 2015) to its series. The ECAD can be used with children ages 2 years, 6 months through age 7 to identify cognitive delays and help determine the need for early intervention. In the spirit of the Woodcock-Johnson tests, the ECAD is based on the contemporary CHC model of intelligence. There are 10 tests included in the measure, which are used to derive three cluster scores. The cluster scores are the General Intellectual Ability-Early Development Cluster, the Early Academic Skills cluster, and the Expressive Language cluster. Further, seven tests comprise the General Intellectual Ability-Early Development cluster, and the three additional tests make up the Early Academic Skills cluster. Two of the former tests are used to calculate the Expressive Language Cluster. The inclusion of the

Early Academic Skills cluster sets the ECAD apart from other preschool tests of cognitive abilities. See Rapid Reference 4.2 for a list of CHC abilities assessed with the ECAD.

The test authors state that the test was designed to include attractive materials that would capture the attention of young children. These materials include a stimulus book and audio recording. No other manipulatives are included in the test, which provides examiners with a convenient and compact assessment kit compared to other options but may not be as appealing to young children as other measures. Although readers may be more familiar with other tests within the Woodcock-Johnson series, the ECAD is highlighted here to introduce readers to this early childhood measure.

Rapid Reference 4.2 Organization of the Tests of Early Cognitive and Academic Development

Cognitive Ability	Test Name
Learning Efficiency (*Gl*)	Memory for Names
Auditory Processing (*Ga*)	Sound Blending
Comprehension-Knowledge (*Gc*)	Picture Vocabulary
Fluid Reasoning (*Gf*)	Verbal Analogies
Visual Processing (*Gv*)	Visual Closure
Short-Term Storage and Working Memory (*Gwm*)	Sentence Repetition
Processing Speed (*Gs*)	Rapid Picture Naming

Achievement Areas	Test Name
Reading	Letter-Word Identification
Mathematics	Number Sense
Written Language	Writing

Sources: V. Alfonso (personal communication, June 11, 2024); Wendling et al. (2015).

***Kaufman Assessment Battery for Children, Second Edition, Normative Update* (KABC-II-NU).** The Kaufman Assessment Battery for Children, Second Edition, Normative Update (KABC-II-NU; Kaufman & Kaufman, 2018) is a measure of cognitive abilities for children and adolescents ages 3–18 years. Initially published in 2004 (Kaufman & Kaufman, 2004), the KABC-II is an attractive choice for examiners when assessing the cognitive abilities of young children due to a normative update in 2018. This normative update allows examiners to continue using previous KABC-II materials with the benefit of having timely norms available to meet the changing make-up of the United States population (Kaufman & Kaufman, 2018). Depending on the age of the child, the KABC-II yields scores on one to five scales and can be interpreted using one of two theoretical models: Luria's Neuropsychological Theory or the CHC model. In most cases, the CHC model is the preferred model of interpretation (Lichtehberger & Kaufman, 2007). When the KABC-II-NU is administered to 3 year olds, only a global scale is obtained. The examiner can choose interpretation through the Nonverbal Index (NVI), the Fluid-Crystallized Index (FCI) or the Mental Processing Index (MPI). Depending on the index chosen, 3 year olds can be administered four to seven core subtests. For ages 4 through 6 years, the KABC-II global index is organized into four CHC components: Short-Term Storage and Working Memory (*Gsm*), Visual Processing (*Gv*), Long-Term Storage and Retrieval/Learning Efficiency (*Glr/Gl*), and Crystallized Ability/Comprehension Knowledge (*Gc*). Four and 5 year olds are administered nine core subtests and 6 year olds are administered 10. Supplemental subtests are also available for this age group. Rapid Reference 4.3 provides descriptions of the core KABC-II NU subtests for the preschool age group and the corresponding CHC broad and narrow abilities that are assessed.

Improving upon the initial version of the KABC-II, the normative update allows for out-of-level testing to better capture the cognitive abilities of young children. Since the age of the child determines the selection of subtests, the addition of out-of-level norms provides more flexibility for the examiner when determining the most appropriate set of subtests for a specific child (Kaufman & Kaufman, 2018). Specifically, the examiner now has the option of administering subtests designed for older or younger children when suspecting a child's cognitive functioning might be higher or lower than his or her peers. The KABC-II-NU includes colorful pictures in the stimulus books, with easy-to-administer subtests that are designed to capture a young child's attention.

≡ Rapid Reference 4.3 Kaufman Assessment Battery for Children, Second Edition, Normative Update, Subtests

CHC Cognitive Ability	Subtest Name
Short-Term Storage and Working Memory (Gsm)	
Auditory Short-Term Storage	Number Recall
Visual–Spatial Short-Term Storage	Word Order
Working Memory Capacity	Word Order
Learning Efficiency (Gl)	
Associative Memory	Atlantis & Rebus
Visual Processing (Gv)	
Visualization	Conceptual Thinking, Pattern Reasoning & Triangles
Visual–Spatial Short-Term Storage	Face Recognition
Spatial Scanning	Rover
Comprehension-Knowledge (Gc)	
Lexical Knowledge	Riddles & Expressive
Language Development	Vocabulary
Mathematical Knowledge	Riddles
	Rover

Sources: From *Kaufman Assessment Battery for Children, Second Edition, Normative Update, Manual Supplement,* by A.S. Kaufman and N.L. Kaufman (2018) & Drozdick et al. (2018). Only core subsets for preschool children are listed. Updated CHC abilities are utilized per V. Alfonso (personal communication, June 11, 2024).

Social–Emotional Skills

Social–emotional skills are a broad set of skills necessary for connecting with others and managing emotions. Consistent with other developmental domains, social–emotional skills follow a predicted developmental trajectory. Young children begin using these skills from birth to connect with caregivers, gain confidence, feel empathy, develop friendships, and manage negative emotions. As discussed later in this chapter, positive social–emotional skills are essential for success in school, so much so that preschools emphasize social skills in the curriculum. The acquisition of these skills, referred to as social–emotional learning (SEL), has become a central aspect of early childhood education (Ellas & Moceri, 2012). In fact, all 50 states have adopted formal social–emotional curriculum for preschool-aged children (Anthony et al., 2020), many adhering to the Collaborative for Academic, Social, and Emotional Learning's framework (Oliver & Berger, 2020). This framework includes addressing young children's skills in the areas of self-awareness, social awareness, responsible decision-making, self-management, and relationship skills. Specifically, social–emotional skills result in the ability to build relationships with others, problem solve in social settings, and cope with stress.

Indicators of well-developed social–emotional functioning include recognizing feelings in self and others, managing emotions, establishing and maintaining relationships, and responsible decision-making, including taking responsibility for one's own actions (Oliver & Berger, 2020). Social–emotional skills are an important component of school readiness; in fact, teachers often place a high value on social–emotional skills for kindergarten readiness (Curby et al., 2017). For example, early childhood educators indicated that cooperation and compliance were two important skills necessary when entering into formal education (Goodrich et al., 2015). Additionally, kindergarten teachers ranked social–emotional skills, such as getting along with others and calming themselves down when upset, as more important than academic skills (Curby et al., 2017). Children who show delays in social–emotional skills may qualify for early intervention or preschool services, making accurate assessment imperative (Whitcomb & Kemp, 2020).

Common ratings scales of social–emotional skills evaluate this domain in two different ways. First, measures may compare the young child to the typical developmental trajectory of prosocial behaviors and skills. When a child falls below expected milestones, data can be used to assist in determining whether a child has a developmental delay in the area of social–emotional development. The Ages and States Questionnaire: Social–Emotional, Second Edition (ASQ:SE-2; Squires et al., 2015), described below, falls under this category of assessment tool. Additionally, assessment measures can help determine if the child engages in problem behaviors that are suggestive of behavioral disorders such as attention deficit hyperactivity disorder, autism spectrum disorder, and anxiety or depressive

> ## DON'T FORGET 4.4
>
> Social–emotional skills are commonly assessed through rating scales. These rating scales can focus on whether a child is meeting appropriate social–emotional milestones, or they can focus on whether a child engages in maladaptive behaviors.

disorders, such as the Behavior Assessment System for Children, Third Edition (BASC-3; Reynolds & Kamphaus, 2015). These two common rating scales used to assess the social–emotional skills of young children are described in the following sections. Several other social–emotional rating scales are available, which are listed in the Appendix.

Ages and Stages Questionnaire: Social–Emotional, Second Edition (ASQ:SE-2)

The Ages and Stages Questionnaire: Social–Emotional, Second Edition (ASQ:SE-2; Squires et al., 2015) assesses social and emotional development of infants and toddlers ages 2–60 months. Although it is only available as a parent-report measure, it is a common screening tool for early detection and referral of developmental behavioral concerns used by daycare centers, preschools, and primary care settings. Multiple studies show evidence for the reliability and validity of the ASQ:SE-2 in measuring the social and emotional development of young children (Briggs et al., 2012; McCrae & Brown, 2018). There is one total score for social–emotional development. The components of that score consist of the child's self-regulation, compliance, social-communication, adaptive functioning, autonomy, affect, and interaction with people.

The ASQ:SE-2 assesses children at nine developmental periods: 2, 6, 12, 18, 24, 30, 36, 48, and 60 months. Parents are asked to rate their child as "often or always," "sometimes," or "rarely or never" engaging in various indicators of appropriate social–emotional development. For example, at 24 months, parents rate their child's sleeping patterns, ability to calm themselves within 15 minutes, use of gestures, interest in toys and other children, and ability to follow simple directions. This norm-based measure included over 14,000 ratings of children in the standardization sample. The ASQ:SE-2 assesses the social and emotional developmental milestones expected at the various ages. Children who fall below the norm-based cut scores should be considered for intervention services if other developmental measures support the need for intervention (Squires et al., 2015). In other words, the ASQ:SE-2 is a viable option that can be used within a comprehensive assessment of developmental skills when determining eligibility for early intervention or preschool services.

Behavior Assessment System for Children, Third Edition (BASC-3)

The Behavior Assessment System for Children, Third Edition (BASC-3; Reynolds & Kamphaus, 2015) is a comprehensive rating scale system that can be used with preschool children. The Preschool Form assesses behavior, emotions, and adaptive functioning of children ages 2 years–5 years, 11 months old and is completed by the child's parent/caregiver (Parent Rating Scale) and/or preschool teacher (Teacher Rating Scale). Specifically, the BASC-3 measures children's adaptive skills, emotional functioning, and problem behaviors in the community, school, and home settings, yielding four composite scores: Adaptive Skills, Behavioral Symptoms, Externalizing Problems, Internalizing Problems. The BASC-3 takes approximately 10–20 minutes to complete, making it a convenient tool to add to a comprehensive assessment of a preschool child. It is important to note that the BASC-3 focuses on the maladaptive and problem behaviors of young children, which are often associated with the most commonly diagnosed behavioral disorders in childhood. These include attention-deficit hyperactivity disorder, oppositional defiant disorder, depressive disorders, anxiety disorders, and autism spectrum disorders (Egger & Angold, 2006). Although a diagnosis of a behavioral disorder is not necessary to determine eligibility for early intervention or preschool services, the BASC-3 provides useful information regarding maladaptive behaviors that could be addressed through a formal intervention plan.

The original BASC was published in Reynolds and Kamphaus (1992) and now includes a Family of Assessments. The BASC-3 offers a Behavioral and Emotional Screening System (BASC-3 BESS), Flex Monitor, and Intervention Guides, which align with the recent emphasis on school-based mental health screening and early intervention for children (Dowdy et al., 2019). In a multitiered system of intervention approach (see Chapter 6 of this volume for more information on this approach), the BASC-3 BESS can be an appropriate screening tool used during Tier I to assess all children for social–emotional and behavioral risk. The BASC-3 Flex Monitor allows school psychologists and other school professionals to monitor a child's progress toward behavioral goals while participating in interventions. It can be used as a curriculum-based measurement tool to monitor the progress of children who have Individualized Education

Programs (IEPs) as progress monitoring is a critical component of these educational plans. The BASC-3 Intervention Guide is designed for the school setting and provides detailed instructions on implementing over 60 behavioral interventions. These interventions can be implemented in the classroom or in small groups and can be facilitated by school counselors, psychologists, or social workers. Additionally, the online scoring platform (i.e., Q-Global) provides the option for examiners to purchase a score report that includes the appropriate intervention strategies based on the behavioral and emotional profile of the individual child. The BASC Family of Assessments is one of the most comprehensive to aid in the assessment to intervention process.

Adaptive Behavior

Adaptive behavior is generally considered a person's independent, autonomous functioning. Edgar Doll is credited as a leader in the assessment of adaptive functioning, especially as it relates to a diagnosis of Intellectual Disability (ID). He believed that the concept of social competence was the most important criterion in establishing a diagnosis of ID (Doll, 1936). Adaptive behavior was described as the skills needed to perform everyday activities with personal independence and within a set of societal expectations. Modern rating scales of adaptive functioning align with these historical concepts and consider the construct as age-dependent, understood within societal norms, and always developing (Saulnier & Klaiman, 2022). In other words, adaptive functioning is what an individual performs independently, appropriate to their age and the norms of their culture. Early childhood adaptive measures often focus on communication skills, self-help skills, interaction with others, and sensorimotor development as reported by a parent, caregiver, and/or teacher. Common methods of assessment include rating scales completed by parents and teachers, interviews conducted by a clinician, and less often, observations of the child directly. Floyd et al. (2015) provide the most recent review of the psychometric properties of adaptive behavior tests used with young children. They conclude that there is an extensive body of evidence supporting the reliability and validity of these tools and indicate that rating scales provided stronger evidence of validity and reliability compared to interview forms (Floyd et al., 2015). Examiners are encouraged to understand the psychometric properties of the tests they select.

Data obtained from adaptive behavior assessments can be used for diagnostic and eligibility purposes, as well as for intervention planning. For instance, if a preschool child has a total adaptive behavior standard score two standard deviations below the mean and displays deficits in their school skills, early childhood educators can create educational goals for the child related to cleaning up art supplies, hanging their coat in their cubby, or attending during circle time for a specified amount of time. As with the other developmental domains, adaptive skills of young children can be assessed through comprehensive developmental measures described later in this chapter. However, many examiners prefer to utilize more comprehensive tools of adaptive functioning such as the Adaptive Behavior Assessment System, Third Edition (ABAS-3; Harrison & Oakland, 2015) and the Vineland Adaptive Behavior Scales, Third Edition (Vineland-3; Sparrow et al., 2016). These measures are described in greater depth in the following sections.

Adaptive Behavior Assessment System, Third Edition (ABAS-3)

The Adaptive Behavior Assessment System, Third Edition (ABAS-3; Harrison & Oakland, 2015) assesses adaptive skills for children and adults from birth to 89 years old. Originally published in 2000, revised in 2003, and again in 2015, the ABAS-3 remains consistent with the adaptive skills included in the diagnostic criteria for Intellectual Developmental Disorder as defined in the *Diagnostic and Statistical Manual of Mental Disorders, Fifth Edition, Text Revision* (DSM-5-TR; American Psychiatric Association, 2022; See Rapid Reference 4.4). Two forms are available for children ages 5 years and under, and these forms can be completed in approximately 15–20 minutes. Parents and caregivers complete the Parent/Primary Caregiver Form for children ages birth to 5 years old and preschool teachers and daycare providers complete the Teacher/Daycare Provider Form for children ages 2–5 years old. If a child is 5 years old, examiners may choose to utilize the Parent or Teacher forms for children ages 5–21. In these cases, the authors of the ABAS-3 suggest that clinicians should choose the birth to 5 forms when the child displays "lower functioning or more severe disabilities, or who have not entered kindergarten," and the 5–21 forms when "for 5-year-old children who are thought to have less severe problems or who have entered kindergarten" (Harrison & Oakland, 2015, p. 10). The ABAS-3 yields a General Adaptive Composite, and Conceptual, Social, and Practical Adaptive Domain standard scores. The Parent/Primary Caregiver and Teacher/Daycare

Provider forms for infants, toddlers, and preschoolers birth to 5 years also include a Motor scaled score that factors into the General Adaptive Composite but not the individual domains.

≡ Rapid Reference 4.4 Adaptive Skill Domains as Identified in the DSM-5-TR

Skill	Definition	Examples
Practical	Behaviors that are used to address personal and health needs.	Taking care of home (such as picking up toys) and functioning in the community.
Conceptual	Behaviors used to accomplish tasks, use academic skills, and communicate with another person.	Competence in memory, language, reading, writing, math reasoning, problem solving, judgment in novel situations.
Social	The ability to have interpersonal interactions, act in a social excepted way, and use leisure time.	Awareness of others' thoughts, feelings, friendship abilities, and social judgment.

Note: These definitions were taken in part from the *Adaptive Behavior Assessment System, Third Edition* (ABAS-3; Harrison & Oakland, 2015) and are the key adaptive areas included in the diagnostic criteria for Intellectual Developmental Disorders as described in the DSM-5-TR (APA, 2022).

Vineland Adaptive Behavior Scales, Third Edition

The Vineland Adaptive Behavior Scales, Third Edition (Vineland-3; Sparrow et al., 2016) assesses adaptive skills of individuals birth to 90 years old. Available in a comprehensive interview form and parent/caregiver and teacher checklists, the Vineland-3 assesses adaptive functioning of young children across the domains of communication, daily living skills, socialization, and motor skills. The Vineland-3 offers brief domain-level versions of each form that yield standard scores across each adaptive area without providing any subdomain scores. These brief forms are available for individuals ages 3 through 21 years and should be used primarily to determine the diagnostic criteria for ID. Although domain scores are available in standard scores, subdomain scores gained from the comprehensive forms are *v-scaled scores* which have a mean of 15 and standard deviation of 3. The Vineland-3 utilized these *v*-scaled scores because they provide for better differentiation at the lower end of functioning (Burger-Caplan et al., 2018), which is useful in determining a functional level for a diagnosis of ID and in determining appropriate interventions. These subdomain scores, however, may be unfamiliar to examiners who do not routinely use the Vineland-3 and may require additional interpretation for stakeholders as they may not be consistent with other scores used in a comprehensive developmental evaluation. Examiners should understand the interpretation of these scores if including the Vineland-3 in their assessment plan.

The Vineland-3 and its predecessors are often described as the most utilized rating scales or surveys of adaptive functioning (Burger-Caplan et al., 2018; Floyd et al., 2015) and much research has been done across all versions. Milne et al. (2020) found that the Vineland-3 accurately identified preschool children in need of substantial support services over another functional measure used in medical settings. Additionally, the Vineland-3 is commonly used in diagnostic evaluations of neurodevelopmental disorders (Bradshaw et al., 2019; Reisinger et al., 2022). When choosing between the interview and rating scale formats of the Vindeland-3, examiners should consider the psychometric properties as well as factors that may impact the interpretation of the results. For instance, research suggests that the rating scale versions of adaptive measures have as good as or better reliability and validity compared to interview versions. Additionally, time-constraints, reading level and language of the informant, and cultural variables may impact the examiner's choice of format.

> **DON'T FORGET 4.5**
>
> The Vineland-3 yields standard scores at the domain level and v-scaled scores at the subdomain level. These subdomain scores may require additional interpretation for stakeholders as they may not be consistent with other scores used in a comprehensive developmental evaluation.

Communication Skills

Speech and language skills fall under the broader category of communication. Communication refers to the exchange of messages between individuals through a variety of means, including speech and verbal and nonverbal language (Caesar & Ottley, 2020). Given the complexity of communication, assessment should occur through a multidisciplinary lens. To determine whether delays in communication skills exist, assessment professionals must first understand typical language development. Although a comprehensive review of typical language development is beyond the scope of this chapter, professionals should understand that speech and language skills progress in a sequential manner. During infancy, babies begin to react to sounds and change their behavior in response to what they hear, and they smile and produce sounds (i.e., babbling) when they are spoken to. As infants progress to toddlers, they move from babbling to using single words. They respond to changes in the tone of an adult's voice, understand the word "no," and attend to a story read to them for a short period of time. Older toddlers follow simple commands, point to pictures when named, and utilize two or more word phrases. More complex communication skills emerge in preschool children. They follow simple directions and answer complex questions. Their vocabularies expand quickly, and they utilize plurals, past-tense verbs, and irregular words (Bornstein & Putnick, 2012). Research has shown that individual differences in language development are stable across the toddler and preschool years (Bornstein & Putnick, 2012). See Rapid Reference 4.5 for examples of speech and language skills typically assessed in a developmental evaluation.

≡ Rapid Reference 4.5 Communication Skills

Skill	Definition	Examples
Speech	This is the ability to communicate with the use of language accurately, clearly, and expressively	
Articulation	Skilled motor behavior that places accurate sounds where they need to be in a word. This is a skill that increases with age.	Child says "seep" for sheep.
Voice	Sound produced by a vocal tract that is made by a specific individual, that can be recognized as that individual.	Tone of voice

Skill	Definition	Examples
Fluency	The successful coordination of motor planning and articulation to string several sounds and words together to create meaning.	Naming several items in a row
Motor Planning	The planning of the sound structure, the order it goes in, and the stress pattern that will be placed on certain syllables.	Coordination of nonword production and sentence production
Language	The combination of understanding what is being said, expressing what they are feeling, and the uncommunicated part of what is happening.	
Expressive	The production and combining of sounds and words to communicate with the world around them.	Speaking and writing
Receptive	The ability to understand what is being spoken.	Listening and reading
Nonverbal	Exchanging emotional status and putting context to the meaning of verbal communication.	Body language, attention, imitation, eye contact, understanding physical gestures, facial expression, and inflections in tone

Note: From Altinkaynak (2019), Canderan et al. (2020), Hamdan (2018), He et al. (2021), Ishikawa et al. (2010), Mailend et al. (2020), Netelenbos et al. (2018), Thurman et al. (2022), Tiwari and Tiwari (2012), Walsh et al. (2015), Yesnazar et al. (2021).

Most language tests assess receptive (i.e., the ability to understand language) and expressive (i.e., the ability to produce sounds and words to communicate) language skills. Communication skills also include pragmatic language skills. Pragmatic language skills refer to the use of language to convey meaning within a context. Similar to overall language impairments, children can exhibit disorders of pragmatic language in the absence of other neurodevelopmental disorders. On the flip side, children with attention deficit hyperactivity disorder, autism spectrum disorder, and language impairments may display difficulty with pragmatic skills (Adams, 2002). Pragmatic language skills in preschool children can be assessed through rating scales and checklists completed by parents, caregivers, and teachers, and formal assessments. In infants and toddlers, structured observations are commonly used and assess for skills such as initiating and responding to joint attention, and social affective and symbolic communication abilities. According to Norbury (2013), the Children's Communication Checklist-2 (CCC-2; Bishop, 2003) is the most widely used checklist to assess pragmatic language skills in children ages 4 through 16 years. Similarly, the Language Use Inventory (O'Neil, 2009) is the only parent-report rating scale to assess early pragmatic language skills in toddlers 18–47 months old. Due to space limitations, an in-depth exploration of these measures is not provided. The reader should consult Bray and deLeyer-Turkes (2023) for a more information on pragmatic skills in young children.

Speech refers to the output of verbal language and is comprised of articulation, voice, and fluency. Motor components tied to speech production include facial and mouth muscles, and muscles of the respiratory system. When speech and language pathologists (SLPs) assess for speech abnormalities in young children, they assess all components that are necessary for the successful production of speech.

SLPs are the primary examiners to measure early speech and language skills in infants, toddlers, and preschool children. Further, SLPs participate in multidisciplinary teams across a variety of settings, including schools, hospitals, and within private clinics. When SLPs are not available, such as in private clinic settings, psychologists are trained to administer and interpret communication assessments so that a comprehensive evaluation of the young child's skills can be completed. In addition to norm-referenced assessment, SLPs often use language sample analysis to compliment standardized test scores. This method allows for a more natural sampling of a child's language and includes data such as mean length of utterance and estimated intelligibility.

Across the United States, preschool children 3–5 years old most commonly qualify for an IEP under the categories of Language Impairment/ Speech Impairment (U.S. Department of Education, 2020). Accurate speech and language assessment leads to the development of appropriate intervention goals. Not only does language assessment lead to accurate eligibility determinations in preschool, but it can be predictive of the young child's skills in other developmental areas. For example, Hohm et al. (2007) found that receptive and expressive language performance at 10 months old was associated with cognitive and academic functioning at 10 years old. Additionally, assessment in infancy was also predictive of verbal and non-verbal communication skills in childhood. Children born pre-term have poorer language outcomes compared to children born at term; however, they may not exhibit atypical articulation patterns (Sanchez et al., 2020). Expressive language skills are associated with behavior problems across the preschool period (Bichay-Awadalla et al., 2020). Furthermore, underdeveloped expressive language skills in boys are related to teacher-reported attention problems in preschool (Zevenbergen & Ryan, 2010). As evident in the literature, language skills in young children are associated with important developmental and behavioral outcomes, underscoring the importance of accurate assessment during infancy, toddlerhood, and the preschool years.

DON'T FORGET 4.6

Speech and language are two distinct areas that fall in the communication domain.

The following sections describe a few common speech and language measures used in the assessment of young children. For a more comprehensive discussion of assessments used in the evaluation of communication skills in young children, see Caesar and Ottley (2020), Sansavini et al. (2021), and Denman et al. (2017).

Receptive Expressive Emergent Language Test, Fourth Edition (REEL-4)

The Receptive Expressive Emergent Language Test, Fourth Edition (REEL-4; Brown et al., 2020) is a caregiver interview measure of the language skills of infants and toddlers birth to 36 months old. The REEL-4 was designed to identify very young children who have language delays or impairments, and to evaluate the language skills of children who have specific disorders that affect language development. The REEL-4 includes a Language Ability composite composed of two subtests, Receptive Language and Expressive Language. It also includes a supplementary Vocabulary Inventory test, which consists of Nouns and Expanded subtests. When norm-referenced assessment of an infant or toddler's language skills cannot be completed, the REEL-4 is a vital tool in a comprehensive developmental evaluation. Independent research using the REEL-4 is limited, but research on previous versions of the REEL indicated standard scores are invariant across gender, minority group status, and speech/language impairment (Hurford & Stutman, 2005).

Preschool Language Scales – Fifth Edition (PLS-5)

The Preschool Language Scales – Fifth Edition (PLS-5; Zimmerman et al., 2011) is the most recent version of the Preschool Language Scales (Zimmerman et al., 1969) that first appeared in 1969 as a measure of language development in young children. Revisions of the PLS (Zimmerman et al., 1979, 1992, 2002, 2011) focused on expanding the language constructs assessed in each version and meeting the need for high-quality assessment measures for infants, toddlers, and preschool children with disabilities (Walker, 1994). Although there are several standardized language tests for use with preschool children (i.e., ages 3–5 years), the PLS-5 is one of only a few direct measures of language comprehension for infants and toddlers (Caesar & Ottley, 2020).

The PLS-5 assesses children from birth to 7 years, 11 months on their comprehensive developmental language. Items range from preverbal, interaction-based items to Theory of Mind and early literacy skills. During the assessment, children point or verbally respond to pictures and objects. Therefore, children who are preverbal can complete this assessment. The assessment provides standard scores for Total Language, Auditory Comprehension, and Expressive Communication. Although norm-referenced assessments are not typically used as progress monitoring tools, the PLS-5 offers Growth Scale Values, which have been shown to be valid indicators of language skill improvement during interventions (Kwok et al., 2022).

Clinical Evaluation of Language Fundamentals-Preschool, Third Edition (CELF Preschool-3)

The Clinical Evaluation of Language Fundamentals-Preschool, Third Edition (CELF Preschool-3; Wiig et al., 2020) is an individualized, comprehensive measure of language and communication skills in young children 3 years–6 years, 11 months old. The original version of the CELF-Preschool was published in 1992 to assess the basic components of language (Wiig et al., 1992). These include semantics morphology, syntax, and auditory memory. The CELF Preschool included six subtests, which yielded a Total Language Score and two language scales, Receptive Language Scale and Expressive Language Scale. Substantial changes have occurred across two revisions, with the CELF Preschool-3 having improved floors and ceilings, modified test items and materials, and additional scaled and index scores to expand the test's scope.

An examiner can obtain a Core Language Score by administering three subtests: Sentence Comprehension, Word Structure, and Expressive Vocabulary. Six additional index scores (Receptive Language Index, Expressive Language Index, Language Content Index, Language Structure Index, Academic Language Readiness Index, and Early Literacy Index) can be calculated from a total of 10 subtests. Although the CELF Preschool-3 can be an important tool for determining eligibility and diagnostic decisions within the language domain, research supports the use of a multi-assessment method (i.e., norm-referenced plus naturalistic assessment) when assessing the language skills of young children (Eadie et al., 2014; Shurman & Leone, 2023).

Goldman-Fristoe Test of Articulation 3 (GFTA-3)

The Goldman-Fristoe Test of Articulation, Third Edition (GFTA-3; Goldman & Fristoe, 2015) assesses articulation and intelligibility of the consonant and consonant cluster sounds of Standard American English for individuals ages 2 years–21 years, 11 months. The test can be used for making educational placements under the category of Speech Impairment or diagnostic decisions of articulation disorders. At young ages, children are asked to name pictures. If the child does not know the word for the picture, the examiner can tell them the name of the picture so that the child can repeat the word. This way, regardless of the young child's vocabulary knowledge, their articulation skills can be assessed. The GFTA-3 provides standard scores in Sounds-In-Words and Sounds-In-Sentences. The child is also scored on their Intelligibility, which is percentage of total intelligibility. Incorrectly articulated sounds or sound clusters at the initial, medial, and final consonant position are noted for intervention planning.

COMPREHENSIVE DEVELOPMENTAL BATTERIES

Evaluation of infant, toddler, and preschool skills often requires comprehensive assessment of all developmental domains. Developmental assessments can be utilized as part of a comprehensive evaluation, or they can be used to screen children to determine in which domain more comprehensive assessment should occur. Depending on the skill level of the infant, toddler, or preschooler, examiners must select the most appropriate tools to gather a comprehensive picture of the child's development. This may include direct measurement of a child's skills through individualized assessment, ratings provided by parents, caregivers, or teachers, observations of the skill by the examiner, or a combination of methods. Although a combination of methods may be the most desirable, examiners must understand the child characteristics, parental skills and limitations, and a variety of uncontrollable environmental factors that may alter the plan at the time of the assessment. Several of these considerations were discussed in Chapter 2 of this volume. Individualized assessment will not always be possible, especially when a young child exhibits an impairment that inhibits the child's ability to perform the task demands of the test. Therefore, developmental rating scales completed by the parent, caregiver, daycare provider, or teacher may be the only reliable and valid measure of a child's skills at the time of assessment.

Administration of comprehensive developmental tests may also depend on the assessment setting. Psychologists in clinical or private settings may take a different approach to a developmental assessment compared to a school psychologist or special education teacher in a school setting. Upon the transition from early intervention into the preschool setting, a multidisciplinary team may utilize one of the comprehensive developmental tools that will be discussed in this chapter, with each team member completing their specific domain of the assessment. For instance, if choosing to complete the Battelle Developmental Inventory, Third Edition (BDI-3; Newborg, 2020a) to assess a 2 year, 11-month-old child, the OT may complete the Fine and Perceptual Motor Subtests. The SLP may then complete the Expressive and Receptive Subtests and the school psychologist may complete subtests within the Cognitive Domain. This same type of assessment plan may occur in an interdisciplinary medical setting as part of a hospital developmental clinic. In a private practice setting, on the other hand, a psychologist may not have access to other service providers. Therefore, the psychologist would likely complete all the subtests in the various developmental domains independently.

Given the complex interconnection of developmental skills in young children, comprehensive developmental measures were designed to evaluate all domains of functioning in one test (Bayley & Aylward, 2019). The following

CAUTION 4.2

Examiners should only administer tests for which they have been trained and are competent to administer.

sections describe two of the most commonly utilized individual developmental measures. Additionally, a comprehensive developmental rating scale and interview system is described as an alternative when individualized testing is not possible.

Bayley Scales of Infant and Toddler Development, Fourth Edition (Bayley-4)

The Bayley Scales of Infant Development (Bayley, 1969) was designed as a developmental measure to assess infant and toddler cognitive abilities, motor skills, and behaviors. Originally published in 1969, it included a Cognitive Scale and Motor Scale. A separate Infant Behavior Record was completed after the assessment to record the behavior of the child during the evaluation. At the time of its publication, few measures appropriate for infants and toddlers assessed multiple developmental domains (Alyward, 1997). The original Bayley assessed infants and toddlers from 2 to 30 months old and was revised in 1993 to update the normative data and expand the age range to 1–42 months old. Further revisions occurred in 2006, which expanded upon the developmental domains assessed by the measure. The Bayley Scales of Infant and Toddler Development, Third Edition (Bayley-III; Bayley, 2006) included five distinct developmental scales: Cognitive, Motor, Language, Social–Emotional, and Adaptive Behavior. The Bayley-III also included modernized items and engaging toys and activities. Updated again in 2019, the revision aimed to simplify administration, include caregivers in the assessment process, and improve the clinical utility of the measure (Bayley & Aylward, 2019). The Bayley Scales of Infant and Toddler Development, Fourth Edition (Bayley-4; Bayley & Aylward, 2019) has been referred to as the "gold-standard" of infant and toddler instruments for developmental assessment and evaluation (Alfonso et al., 2022) and can be administered to infants and toddlers 1–42 months old.

Retained from the Bayley-III, the Bayley-4 consists of five developmental scales: Cognitive, Language, Motor, Social–Emotional, and Adaptive Behavior. The Cognitive, Motor, and Language Scales include structured items for direct assessment of skills. Language assessment is further divided into Receptive Communication and Expressive Communication subtests, and the Motor composite consists of Fine Motor and Gross Motor subtests. Parents and caregivers should be present during assessment of these scales to provide insight into the young child's behaviors outside of the assessment setting. Caregivers also complete the Social–Emotional and Adaptive Behavior Scales via a questionnaire format. The Adaptive Behavior Scale consists of Communication, Daily Living Skills, and Socialization Domains. It is important to note that the Bayley-4 does not include one overall score of development due to the interconnectedness of the infant and toddler development (Bayley & Aylward, 2019). See Alfonso et al. (2022) for a thorough discussion of the Bayley-4.

Battelle Developmental Inventory, Third Edition (BDI-3)

The Battelle Developmental Inventory (BDI) was originally published in 1984 to assess the developmental trajectory of infants and toddlers in the Adaptive, Personal-Social, Communication, Motor, and Cognitive developmental domains (Alfonso et al., 2010). The Battelle Developmental Inventory, Third Edition (BDI-3; Newborg, 2020a) is the latest iteration of the popular developmental test used to assess infants and toddlers from birth to 95 months (7 years, 11 months) old. Compared to previous iterations, the BDI-3 uses fewer manipulatives for easier administration. Published by Riverside, the BDI-3 can be administered and scored via the Riverside Score Mobile Solutions data app. Traditional administration and hand scoring are also available. Designed to meet federal assessment guidelines under IDEA (2004) and Head Start programming, assessment results from the BDI-3 can aid in the development of Individualized Family Service Plan (IFSP) and IEP goals. Intended to identify children with developmental delays or advanced development, the test publisher cautions against using the BDI-3 as a diagnostic tool to identify disorders such as intellectual disabilities or attention deficit hyperactivity disorder.

The BDI-3 yields five domain standard scores (Adaptive, Social–Emotional, Communication, Motor, and Cognitive), with each domain comprised of two to three subdomains. If all domains are administered to the child, a BDI-3 Total Developmental Quotient Score can be obtained. Examiners can select relevant domains for administration during an evaluation based on the referral question. Items across the 13 subdomains vary in administration procedure. Some items require structured administration; others can be scored through direct observation of the skill during the assessment; and lastly, item scores can also be obtained through interview with the parent or caregiver. The stimulus books and record form indicate which administration procedure is appropriate for each item, and the examiner should note in the appropriate section of the record form which procedure was used. Structured administration requires standardized procedures in a controlled, one-on-one setting, whereas items coded as interview can be obtained through parent or caregiver report. Examiners should be aware of all appropriate administration procedures, but structured administration is preferred if presented as an option.

Developmental Profile 4 (DP4)

The Developmental Profile 4 (DP4; Alpern, 2020) allows for the assessment of individuals birth through 21 years 11 months old across multiple settings. Encompassing the developmental domains included in the IDEA eligibility, the DP4 has multiple forms to gain the most comprehensive data through multiple assessment methods and informants. Results from the DP4 can be utilized to identify strengths and weaknesses of the child, assist in determining special education eligibility, and assist in writing intervention goals. Adding the DP4 to a developmental assessment has several benefits. First, the DP4 allows for comparisons across teacher and parent/caregiver ratings. Second, the DP4 provides growth scores which allows examiners to compare progress over time. Third, the DP4 can be utilized to obtain an estimate of a child's functioning across the various developmental domains when conducting a remote assessment (Jang et al., 2022). Fourth, the DP4 allows examiners to obtain a comprehensive view of a child's skills with one assessment. Finally, the DP4 gathers a lot of information in a short amount of time. For example, when young children struggle to participate in a lengthy individualized assessment, parents can complete one checklist or interview to determine their child's functional level. The ability to obtain standard scores across all five developmental domains without the need for direct assessment makes the DP4 an ideal tool during a multidisciplinary evaluation.

The DP4 forms include parent/caregiver and teacher checklists, a parent/caregiver interview, and a checklist completed by the examiner. Since these forms are not individually administered with the child, ratings represent the respondent's perception of the child, not necessarily what they can and cannot do. The Physical Scale assesses fine and gross motor skills. The Adaptive Behavior Scale assesses daily-living skills such as self-care, eating, dressing, and accessing modern technology. The Social–Emotional Scale assesses the child's ability to relate to others and function within a social setting. At the young ages, the Cognitive Scale assesses

DON'T FORGET 4.7

Parents, caregivers, and teachers can provide perspective on the child's developmental skills through an interview or checklist format, like those available with the DP4, when standardized testing cannot be conducted or completed.

skills that are prerequisite skills for successful academic performance. Finally, the Communication Scale encompasses expressive and receptive language and verbal and non-verbal communication skills. Standard scores are obtained across these areas, which align with the IDEA developmental domains.

FUNCTIONAL PREACADEMICS

School readiness is commonly conceptualized as a child's acquired preacademic skills prior to kindergarten; however, this concept is much more complex. Some researchers define it as a maturational process where a child naturally develops the necessary skills seen as important for entry into kindergarten, whereas others see it as a set of skills that are taught through culture (Hojnoski & Missall, 2020). Despite these varying viewpoints, research suggests that child competencies (i.e., their developmental skills) are strongly associated with early academic success (Romano et al., 2010). For instance, Lin and colleagues (2003) surveyed over 3,000 kindergarten teachers and found that the school readiness was strongly tied to the social aspects of learning. These findings persist despite the shift to a more academic focus in kindergarten in school in the United States. Studies have found that kindergarten teachers continue to rate nonacademic factors (e.g., getting along with others, sharing, understanding emotions, and calming themselves when upset) as the most important aspect of kindergarten readiness (Curby et al., 2017; Hustedt et al., 2018). This research highlights the importance of assessing both academic and nonacademic domains of kindergarten readiness in young children. The following section focuses on the assessment of functional preacademic skills, which is only one component of school readiness.

Foundational skills in reading, math, and writing have been linked to later academic success (Manfra et al., 2017). These skills include being able to hold a pencil, draw lines, draw figures and letters, count, identify letters and their corresponding sounds, recognize patterns, and persist with challenging tasks. During early childhood, foundational literacy skills teach the child to interact with the world through writing and print media (i.e., books). Literacy skills begin with parents reading to their children from a young age. Foundational math skills include shape and pattern identification as well as numbers and counting. Once young children can count, they then often learn to identify "how many" of an object are present (Geary & vanMarle, 2018). The assessments described below focus on evaluating a young child's knowledge in these pre-academic areas; however, the literature identifies other foundational academic skills that are important for success (Cameron et al., 2012; McDermott et al., 2014). These include the concept of a child's approach to learning, which encompasses their skills at building cognitive, behavioral, and emotional self-regulation, as well as their curiosity for learning and creativity. Motor skills are also considered an important foundational skill that is associated with later academic success. A thorough discussion of all the concepts related to kindergarten readiness is beyond the scope of this chapter; therefore, the following sections focus on assessments of preacademic skills.

DON'T FORGET 4.8

Foundational skills refer to the building blocks of reading, math, and writing skills, which have been linked to later academic success.

Bracken Basic Concept Scale (BBCS) and Bracken School Readiness Assessment, Fourth Edition (BSRA-4)

Bracken described school readiness as the understanding of basic concepts and vocabulary necessary to comprehend classroom instructions and communication (Bracken & Panter, 2011). In 1984, he developed the Bracken Basic Concept Scale (BBCS; Bracken, 1984) to assess basic vocabulary concepts within a categorical schema necessary for all young children to understand before entering formal education. This initial edition assessed the receptive understanding of basic concepts across 11 domains: Colors, Letters, Numbers/Counting, Sizes, Shapes, Comparisons, Direction/Position, Self-/Social-Awareness, Texture/Material, Quantity, and Time/Sequence. The BBCS was revised and renormed in 1997, and again in 2007 when it was divided into separate expressive and receptive scales in response to practitioners need for assessment in both areas to help drive targeted intervention (Bracken & Panter, 2011). The receptive scale was updated in 2022 and provides School Readiness Composite and Receptive Total Composite standard scores and up to 10 subtest scaled scores.

The Bracken School Readiness Assessment (BSRA; Bracken, 2002) is a separate scale comprised of the School Readiness Composite from the BBCS and is commonly used to screen for kindergarten readiness. Many studies have supported the validity of the BSRA in predicting later cognitive and academic abilities (see Panter & Bracken, 2009). The Bracken School Readiness Assessment, Fourth Edition (BSRA-4; Bracken, 2022) systematically assesses concepts often taught in early childhood educational programs. It includes foundational academic skills in the areas of Colors, Letters, Numbers/Counting, Sizes/Comparison, and Shapes. This newest version added one subtest called Self-/Social Awareness, expanding the previous version's conceptualization of school-readiness to match the nonacademic components found in the literature (i.e., Hustedt et al., 2018). Additionally, more items were added to improve the floor and ceiling of the test. The BSRC-4 is an easy-to-administer assessment that can be completed in 15–20 minutes by a trained examiner. It consists of several features necessary when assessing young children such as being colorful to maintain attention and having updated norms.

Battelle Early Academic Survey

The Battelle Early Academic Survey (BEAS; Newborg, 2020b) is an individually administered survey of foundational academic skills in the areas of literacy and mathematics. Designed as a screening tool or survey, the BEAS helps identify children, ages 3 years 6 months–7 years 11 months, who are at risk for delays in these academic areas. According to the examiner's manual, administration of the BEAS should take approximately 35–45 minutes, depending on the age and the skill level of the child. Children with developmental delays often struggle with the development of preacademic skills, and the BEAS was designed as a companion tool to the BDI-3 to assist developmental specialists in understanding the comprehensive skill set of a child who may need interventions. The survey yields domain and subdomain scores across the areas of Literacy and Mathematics. The Literacy Domain contains five subdomains, including Print Concepts, Phonological Awareness, Phonics and Word Recognition, Listening Comprehension, and Fluency. To provide the reader with an idea of the comprehensive nature of the pre-academic skills assessed with the BEAS, Rapid Reference 4.6 includes a description of each subdomain/ area assessed in the Literacy Domain of the BEAS.

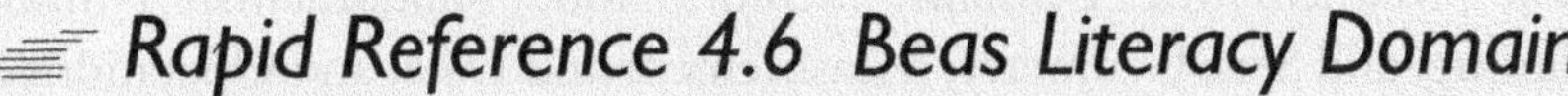 Rapid Reference 4.6 Beas Literacy Domain

Subdomain/Area	Skills Measured
Print Concepts	Demonstrate an understanding of basic print concepts while looking at a book
Phonological Awareness	
Rhyming	Identify rhyming and nonrhyming words
Syllables	Break syllables into words; blend syllables to make words
Onset Rime	Identify initial sounds in words; blend initial sounds with word parts to create whole words
Phoneme Identification	Identify phonemes in initial, medial, and ending portions within words
Phoneme Blending and Segmenting	Blend individual phonemes to create words; break words into individual phonemes
Phoneme Manipulation	Add and remove phonemes in the initial and ending positions in words; substitute phonemes in the initial medial, and ending position to create new words
Phonics and Word Recognition	
Letter Identification	Identify uppercase and lowercase letters presented visually
Letter-Sound Correspondence	Produce sounds corresponding to letters presented visually
Early Decoding	Match pictures with consonant-vowel-consonant words
Sight Words	Read sight words aloud
Nonsense Words	Apply phonetic decoding skills to read nonsense words
Long Vowel Patterns	Apply knowledge of long and short vowel patterns to match pictures with words
Inflectional Endings	Identify the correct word in a series based on an understanding of inflectional endings
Listening Comprehension	Answer questions pertaining to short passages and stories presented orally
Fluency	Timed. Correctly name pictures of familiar objects under a timed condition

Source: Adapted from BEAS Examiner's Manual Newborg (2020b).

The Mathematics Domain includes four subdomains: Numbers, Counting, and Sets; Geometry; Measurement and Data; and Operations and Algebraic Thinking. These subdomains measure skills such as counting using one-to-one correspondence, labeling shapes, completing patterns, telling time, and simple addition and subtraction problems. Given the comprehensive nature of many of the skills assessed in this measure, examiners must understand the developmental level of the preschooler when selecting the appropriate preacademic measure.

SUMMARY

This chapter focused on assessment across the IDEA developmental domains. Consistent with federal law (i.e., IDEA), infants, toddlers, and preschoolers suspected of developmental differences should be assessed in a comprehensive manner. This requires examiners to assess the five areas of development contained in federal law: physical development, cognitive development, communication development, social or emotional development, and adaptive development. Assessment of young children can be done by utilizing developmental tests that encompass all domains. Assessment can also be accomplished at the individual or specific domain level with separate tests and integrating the data to form a comprehensive evaluation of the young child. Regardless of the manner, reliable and valid assessment of developmental skills is vital for the creation of appropriate IFSP or IEP goals and intervention planning.

TEST YOURSELF

1. **IDEA references all of the following developmental areas except:**
   (a) Cognitive abilities
   (b) Preacademic skills
   (c) Motor skills
   (d) Social and emotional skills
2. **Which of the following is a direct measurement of a child's skills:**
   (a) Ratings completed by caregivers
   (b) Observations of skill by assessment specialist
   (c) Individualized assessment
   (d) All the above

3. **Which subtest on Bracken School Readiness Composite, Fourth Edition is new to this updated version:**
   (a) Colors
   (b) Number/Counting
   (c) Self-/Social Awareness
   (d) Letters

4. **The Battelle Developmental Inventory, Third Edition was not designed to help with establishing what kind of goals?**
   (a) Individualized Family Service Plans
   (b) Individualized Education Plans
   (c) Impact of Medication
   (d) All the above

5. **Which of the following is a characteristic provided by the Developmental Profile 4:**
   (a) A comprehensive view of a child's skills with one assessment
   (b) Examiners observe the child's skills by having children perform tasks for them
   (c) There is a self-report option for when the child reaches a certain age
   (d) All the above

6. **Infant cognitive abilities are influenced by which of the following factors?**
   (a) Birth weight
   (b) Access to play materials at home
   (c) Motor skills
   (d) All of the above

7. **The Woodcock-Johnson IV Tests of Early Cognitive and Academic Development align with which model of intelligence?**
   (a) Cattell-Horn-Carroll
   (b) General Intelligence
   (c) Primary Mental Abilities
   (d) Multiple Intelligences

8. **What is the benefit of the Kaufman Assessment Battery for Children, Second Edition, Normative Update?**
   (a) Examiners can continue using KABC-II materials but with new norms
   (b) The norms were expanded to include more diverse populations and are more representative of the global population
   (c) The norms now align with the General Intelligence model
   (d) There was no benefit

9. Personal and health skills fall under which adaptive behavior domain?

(a) Conceptual

(b) Practical

(c) Social

(d) None of the above

10. An examiner asks a child to name as many fruits as they can in one minute. What skill of speech is the examiner assessing?

(a) Articulation

(b) Voice

(c) Fluency

(d) Motor Planning

Answers: 1. b; 2. d; 3. c; 4. c; 5. a; 6. d; 7. a; 8. a; 9. b; 10. c

REFERENCES

Adams, C. (2002). Practitioner review: The assessment of language pragmatics. *Journal of Child Psychology and Psychiatry, 43,* 973–987. https://doi.org/10.1111/1469-7610.00226

Alfonso, V. C., Engler, J. R., & Turner, A. D. (2022). *Essentials of Bayley-4 assessment.* Wiley.

Alfonso, V. C., Rentz, E. A., & Chung, S. (2010). Review of the Battelle developmental inventory, second edition. *Journal of Early Childhood & Infant Psychology, 6,* 21–40.

Alpern, G. D. (2020). *Developmental profile 4.* WPS.

Altinkaynak, S. Ö. (2019). Investigation of the relationship between parental attitudes and children's receptive and expressive language skills. *Online Submission, 7*(3), 892–903.

Alyward, G. P. (1997). Conceptual issues in developmental screening and assessment. *Journal of Developmental & Behavioral Pediatrics, 18*(5), 340–349. https://doi.org/10.1097/00004703-199710000-00010

Alyward, G. P. (2002). Cognitive and neuropsychological outcomes: More than just IQ scores. *Developmental Disabilities Research Reviews, 8*(4), 234–240. https://doi.org/10.1002/mrdd.10043

American Psychiatric Association. (2022). *Diagnostic and statistical manual of mental disorders* (5th ed., Text Revision). Author.

Anthony, C. J., Elliot, S. N., DiPerna, J. C., & Lei, P. (2020). Multirater assessment of young children's social and emotional learning via the SIS SEL Brief Scales – Preschool Forms. *Early Childhood Research Quarterly, 53,* 625–637. https://doi.org/10.1016/j.ecresq.2020.07.006

Ayres, A. J. (2005). *Sensory integration and the child.* Western Psychological Services.

Bayley, N. (1969). *The Bayley scales of infant development.* Psychological Corporation.

Bayley, N. (2006). *Bayley scales of infant and toddler development* (3rd ed.: Administration manual). Harcourt.

Bayley, N., & Aylward, G. P. (2019). *Bayley-4: Scales of infant and toddler development* (4th ed. [technical manual]). Pearson.

Beery, K. E., & Beery, N. A. (2010). *The Beery-Buktenica developmental test of visual-motor integration* (6th ed.). Pearson Clinical Assessment.

Bichay-Awadalla, K., Qi, C. H., Bulotsky-Shearer, R. J., & Carta, J. J. (2020). Bidirectional relationship between language skills and behavior problems in preschool children from low-income families. *Journal of Emotional and Behavioral Disorders*, *28*(2), 114–128. https://doi.org/10.1177/1063426619853535

Bishop, D. V. M. (2003). *Children's communication checklist-2.* Psychologist Corporation.

Bornstein, M. H., & Putnick, D. L. (2012). Stability of language in childhood: A multiage, multidomain, multimeasure, and multisource study. *Developmental Psychology*, *48*, 477–491. https://doi.org/10.1037/a0025889

Bracken, B. A. (1984). *Bracken basic concept scale.* NCS Pearson.

Bracken, B. A. (2002). *Bracken school readiness assessment.* The Psychological Corporation.

Bracken, B. A. (2022). *Bracken school readiness assessment* (4th ed.). Pearson.

Bracken, B. A., & Panter, J. E. (2011). Using the Bracken basic concept scale and Bracken development program in the assessment and remediation of young children's concept development. *Psychology in the Schools*, *48*, 464–475. https://doi.org/10.1002/pits.20568

Bradshaw, J., Gillespie, S., Klaiman, C., Klin, A., & Saulnier, C. (2019). Early emergence of discrepancy in adaptive behavior and cognitive skills in toddlers with autism spectrum disorder. *Autism*, *23*, 1485–1496. https://doi.org/10.1177/1362361318815662

Bray, M., & deLeyer-Turkes, J. (2023). Best practices in the assessment of children's communication disorders. In P. Harrison, S. Proctor, & A. Thomas (Eds) Best Practices in School Psychology, Seventh Edition. National Association of School Psychologists.

Briggs, R. D., Stettler, E. M., Silver, E. J., Schrag, R. D. A., Nayak, M., Chinitz, S., & Racine, A. D. (2012). Social-emotional screening for infants and toddlers in primary care. *Pediatrics*, *129*(3). https://doi.org/10.1542/peds.2010-2211

Brown, T., Almiento, L., Yu, M., & Bhopti, A. (2023). The sensory processing measure – second edition: A critical review and appraisal. *Occupational Therapy in Health Care*, *38*, 1–34. https://doi.org/10.1080/07380577.2023.2280216

Brown, V. L., Bzoch, K. R., & League, R. (2020). *REEL-4: Receptive-expressive emergent language test* (3rd ed.). Pro-Ed.

Brown, T., Swayn, E., & Marmol, J. M. P. (2021). The relationship between children's sensory processing and executive functions: An exploratory study. *Journal of Occupational Therapy, Schools & Early Intervention*, *14*, 307–324. https://doi.org/10.1080/19411243.2021.1875386

Burger-Caplan, R., Saulnier, C. A., & Sparrow, S. S. (2018). Vineland adaptive behavior scales. In J. S. Kreutzer, J. DeLuca, & B. Caplan (Eds.), *Encyclopedia of Clinical Neuropsychology*. Springer. https://doi.org/10.1007/978-3-319-57111-9_1602

Caesar, L. G., & Ottley, S. W. (2020). Assessing communication, language, and speech in preschool children. In V. C. Alfonso, B. A. Bracken, & R. J. Nagle (Eds.), *Psychoeducational assessment of preschool children* (5th ed., pp. 250–282). Routledge.

Cameron, C. E., Brock, L. L., Murrah, W. M., Bell, L. H., Worzalla, S. L., Grissmer, D., & Morrison, F. L. (2012). Fine motor skills and executive function both contribute to kindergarten achievement. *Child Development*, *83*(4), 1229–1244. https://doi.org/10.1111/j.1467-8624.2012.01768.x

Camerota, M., Gueron-Sela, N., Grimes, M., & Propper, C. B. (2020). Longitudinal links between maternal factors and infant cognition: Moderation by infant sleep. *Infancy*, *25*(2). https://doi.org/10.1111/infa.12321

Canderan, C., Maieron, M., Fabbro, F., & Tomasino, B. (2020). Understanding body language does not require matching the body's egocentric map to body posture: A brain activation fMRI study. *Perceptual & Motor Skills*, *127*(1), 8–35. https://doi.org/10.1080/17405629.2020.1789860

Carlson, A. G., Rowe, E., & Curby, T. W. (2013). Disentangling fine motor skills' relations to academic achievement: The relative contributions of visual spatial integration and visual motor coordination. *The Journal of Genetic Psychology, 175*(5), 514–533. https://doi.org/10.1080/00221325.2012.717122

Centers for Disease Control and Prevention. (2021). Developmental milestones. Retrieved April 24, 2024 from https://www.cdc.gov/ncbddd/actearly/pdf/FULL-LIST-CDC_LTSAE-Checklists2021_Eng_FNL2_508.pdf.

Coallier, M., Rouleau, N., Bara, F., & Morin, M. F. (2014). Visual-motor skills performance on the Beery-VMI: A study of Canadian kindergarten children. *The Open Journal of Occupational Therapy, 2*(2), 4.

Curby, T. W., Berke, E., Alfonso, V. C., Blake, J., DeMarie, D., DuPaul, G. J., Flores, R., Hess, R. S., Howard, K., Lepore, J., & C., & Subotnik, R. F. (2017). Kindergarten teacher perceptions of kindergarten readiness: The important of social-emotional skills. *Perspectives on Early Childhood Psychology and Education, 2*(2), 115–137.

Dale, B. A., Caemmerer, J. M., Winter, E. L., & Kaufman, A. S. (2022). Bayley-4 performance of very young children with autism, developmental delay, and language impairment. *Psychology in the Schools, 59*, 1267–1281. https://doi.org/10.1002/pits.22682

D'Costa, A. G., & Hanig, K. M. (2014). Test of Visual-Motor Skills–3rd Edition. *The Nineteenth Mental Measurements Yearbook.*

Denman, D., Speyer, R., Munro, N., Pearce, W. M., Chen, Y., & Cordier, R. (2017). Psychometric properties of language assessments for children aged 4—12 years: A systematic review. *Frontiers in Psychology, 8*, 1–28. https://doi.org/10.3389/fpsyg.2017.01515

Doll, E. A. (1936). Idiot, imbecile, and moron. *Journal of Applied Psychology, 20*(4), 427–437. https://doi.org/10.1037/h0056577

Dourou, E., Komessariou, A., Riga, V., & Lavidas, K. (2017). Assessment of gross and fine motor skills in preschool children using the Peabody Developmental Motor Scales Instrument. *European Psychomotricity Journal, 9*, 89–113.

Dowdy, E., DiStefano, C., Greer, F., Moore, S., & Pompey, K. (2019). Examining the latent structure of the BASC-3 BESS parent preschool form. *Journal of Psychoeducational Assessment, 37*(2), 181–193. https://doi.org/10.1177/0734282917739109

Drozdick, L. W., Singer, J. K., Lichtenberger, E. O., Kaufman, J. C., Kaufman, A. S., & Kaufman, N. L. (2018). The Kaufman assessment battery for children—Second edition and KABC-II normative update. In D. P. Flanagan & E. M. McDonough (Eds.), *Contemporary intellectual assessment: Theories, tests, and issues* (4th ed.). The Guilford Press.

Dunn, W. (1999). *Sensory profile* (pp. 317–342). Psychological Corporation.

Dunn, W. (2007). Supporting children to participate successfully in everyday life by using sensory processing knowledge. *Infants & Young Children, 20*(2), 84–101. https://doi.org/10.1097/01.IYC.0000264477.05076.5d

Dunn, W. (2014). *Sensory Profile—2.* NSC Pearson.

Eadie, P., Nguyen, C., Carlin, J., Bavin, E., Bretherton, L., & Riley, S. (2014). Stability of language performance at 4 and 5 years: Measurement and participant variability. *International Journal of Language and Communication Disorders, 49*(2), 215–227. https://doi.org/10.1111/1460-6984.12065

Eeles, A., Spittle, A. J., Anderson, P. J., Brown, N., Lee, K. J., Boyd, R. N., Doyle, L., & W. (2013). Assessments of sensory processing in infants: A systematic review. *Developmental Medicine and Child Neurology, 55*, 296–392. https://doi.org/10.1111/j1469-8749.2012.04434.x

Egger, H. L., & Angold, A. (2006). Common emotional and behavioral disorders in preschool children: Presentation, nosology, and epidemiology. *Journal of Child Psychology and Psychiatry, 47*, 313–337. https://doi.org/10.1111/j.1469-7610.2006.01618.x

Ellas, M. J., & Moceri, D. C. (2012). Developing social and emotional aspects of learning: The American experience. *Research Papers in Education, 27*, 423–434. https://doi.org/10.1080/02671522.2012.690243

Engler, J. R., & Alfonso, V. C. (2020). Cognitive assessment of preschool children: A pragmatic review of theoretical, quantitative, and qualitative characteristics. In V. C. Alfonso, B. A. Bracken, & R. J. Nagle (Eds.), *Psychoeducational assessment of preschool children* (5th ed., pp. 226–249). Routledge.

Estaki, M., Dehghan, A., Kojidi, E. M., & Mirzakhany, N. (2021). Psychometric evaluation of the child sensory profile 2 (CSP2) among children with dyslexia. *Iran Journal of Behavioral Science, 15*, 1–7. https://doi.org/10.5812/ijpbs.112573

Feeding Matters. (2024). What is PFD? Retrieved January 5, 2024 from https://www.feedingmatters.org/what-is-pfd/.

Ferretti, L. K., & Bub, K. L. (2017). Family routines and school readiness during the transition to kindergarten. *Early Education and Development, 28*, 59–77. https://doi.org/10.1080/10409289.2016.1195671

Field, S., Esposito Bosma, C. B., & Temple, V. A. (2020). Comparability of the test of gross motor development-second edition and the test of gross motor development-third edition. *Journal of Motor Learning and Development, 8*, 107–125. https://doi.org/10.1123/jmld.2018-0058

Floyd, R. G., Shands, E. I., Alfonso, V. C., Phillips, J. F., Autry, B. K., Mosteller, J. A., Skinner, M., & Irby, S. (2015). Systematic review and psychometric evaluation of adaptive behavior scales and recommendations for practice. *Journal of Applied School Psychology, 31*, 83–113. https://doi.org/10.1080/15377903.2014.979384

Folio, M., & Fewell, R. (2000). *Peabody developmental motor scales (PDMS-2)*. Pro-Ed.

Geary, D. C., & vanMarle, K. (2018). Growth of symbolic number knowledge accelerates after children understand cardinality. *Cognition, 177*, 69–78. https://doi.org/10.1016/j.cognition.2018.04.002

Goday, P. S., Huh, S. Y., Silverman, A., Lukens, C. T., Dodrill, P., Cohen, S. S., Delaney, L., Feuling, M. B., Noel, R. J., Gisel, E., Kenzer, A., Kessler, D. B., de Camargo, O. K., Browne, J., & Phalen, J. A. (2019). Pediatric feeding disorder: Consensus definition and conceptual framework. *Journal of Pediatric Gastroenterology and Nutrition, 68*, 124–129. https://doi.org/10.1097/MPG.0000000000002188

Goldman, R., & Fristoe, M. (2015). *Goldman fristoe test of articulation 3*. NCS Pearson.

Goodrich, S., Mudrick, H., & Robinson, J. (2015). The transition from early child care to preschool: Emerging skills and readiness for group-based learning. *Early Education and Development, 26*, 1035–1056. https://doi.org/10.1080/10409289.2015.1006978

Goodway, J. D., Robinson, L. E., & Crowe, H. (2010). Gender differences in fundamental motor skill development in disadvantaged preschoolers from two geographical regions. *Research Quarterly for Exercise and Sport, 81*(1), 17–24.

Hamdan, M. A. (2018). Developing a proposed training program based on discrete trial training (DTT) to improve the non-verbal communication skills in children with autism spectrum disorder (ASD). *International Journal of Special Education, 33*(3), 579–591.

Hardy, L. L., King, L., Farrell, L., Macniven, R., & Howlett, S. (2010). Fundamental movement skills among Australian preschool children. *Journal of Science and Medicine in Sport, 13*, 503–508. https://doi.org/10.1016/j.jsams.2009.05.010

Harrison, P. L., & Oakland, T. (2015). *Adaptive behavior assessment system* (3rd ed. [Manual]). Western Psychological Services.

He, J., Meyer, A. S., & Brehm, L. (2021). Concurrent listening affects speech planning and fluency: The roles of representational similarity and capacity limitation. *Language, Cognition and Neuroscience, 36*(10), 1258–1280. https://doi.org/10.1080/23273798.2021.1925130

Hendry, A., Gibson, S. P., Davies, C., Gliga, T., McGillion, M., & Gonzalez-Gomez, N. (2022). Not all babies are in the same boat: Exploring the effects of socioeconomic status, parental attitudes, and activities during the 2020 COVID-19 pandemic on early executive functions. *Journal of the International Congress of Infant Studies, 27*, 555–581. https://doi.org/10.1111/infa.12460

Hohm, E., Jennen-Steinmetz, C., Schmidt, M. H., & Laucht, M. (2007). Language development at ten months: Predictive of language outcome and school achievement ten years later? *European Journal of Child and Adolescent Psychiatry, 16,* 149–156. https://doi.org/10.1007/s00787-006-0567-y

Hojnoski, R. L., & Missall, K. N. (2020). School readiness and academic functioning in preschoolers. In V. C. Alfonso, B. A. Bracken, & R. J. Nagle (Eds.), *Psychoeducational assessment of preschool children* (5th ed., pp. 79–97). Routledge.

Hurford, D. P., & Stutman, G. (2005). *Receptive-expressive emergent language test* (3rd ed.). The Sixteenth Mental Measurements Yearbook.

Hustedt, J. T., Buell, M. J., Hallam, R. A., & Pinder, W. M. (2018). While kindergarten has changed, some beliefs stay the same: Kindergarten teachers' beliefs about readiness. *Journal of Research in Childhood Education, 32*(1), 52–66. https://doi.org/10.1080/02568543.2017.1393031

IDEA. (2004). Individuals with Disabilities Education Improvement Act [IDEA] of 2004, 20 U.S.C 1400 et seq.

Ishikawa, H., Hashimoto, H., Kinoshita, M., & Yano, E. (2010). Can nonverbal communication skills be taught? *Medical Teacher, 32*(10), 860–863. https://doi.org/10.3109/01421591003728211

Jang, J., White, S. P., Esler, A. N., Kim, S. H., Klaiman, C., Megerian, J. T., Morse, A., Nadler, C., & Kanne, S. M. (2022). Diagnostic evaluations of autism spectrum disorder during the COVID-19 pandemic. *Journal of Autism and Developmental Disorders, 52,* 962–973. https://doi.org/10.1007/s10803-021-04960-7

Jorquera-Cabrera, S., Romero-Ayuso, D., Rodriguez-Gil, G., & Trivino-Juarez, J. (2017). Assessment of sensory processing characteristics in children between 3 and 11 years old: A systematic review. *Frontiers in Pediatrics, 5,* 1–18. https://doi.org/10.3389/fped.2017.00057

Kaufman, A. S., & Kaufman, N. L. (2004). *Kaufman assessment battery for children—Second edition (KABC-II) [Manual].* Pearson.

Kaufman, A. S., & Kaufman, N. L. (2018). *Kaufman assessment battery for children* (2nd ed. Normative Update). NCS Pearson.

Kerr-Wilson, C. O., Mackay, D. F., Smith, G. C. S., & Pell, J. P. (2012). Meta-analysis of the association between preterm delivery and intelligence. *Journal of Public Health, 34*(2), 209–216. https://doi.org/10.1093/pubmed/fdr024

Klein-Radukic, S., & Zmyj, N. (2023). The predictive value of the cognitive scale of the Bayley Scales of Infant and Toddler Development-III. *Cognitive Development, 65,* 101291. https://doi.org/10.1016/j.cogdev.2022.101291

Kokstejn, J., Musalek, M., & Tufano, J. J. (2017). Are sex differences in fundamental motor skills uniform throughout the entire preschool period? *PLoS One, 12*(4), e0176556. https://doi.org/10.1371/journal.pone.0176556

Kovacic, K., Rein, L. E., Kommareddy, S., Bhagavatula, P., & Goday, P. S. (2020). Pediatric feeding disorder: A nationwide prevalence study. *Journal of Pediatrics, 228,* 126–131. https://doi.org/10.1016/j.jpeds.2020.07.047

Kwok, E., Feiner, H., Grauzer, J., Kaat, A., & Roberts, M. Y. (2022). Measuring change during intervention using norm-referenced standardized measures: A comparison of raw scores, standard scores, age equivalents, and growth scale values from the Preschool Language Scales – Fifth Edition. *Journal of Speech, Language, and Hearing, 65,* 4268–4279. https://doi.org/10.1044/2022_JSLHR-22-00122

Licciardi, L., & Borwn, T. (2023). An overview & critical review of the Sensory Profile—second edition. *Scandinavian Journal of Occupational Therapy, 30,* 758–770. https://doi.org/10.1080/11038128.2021.1930148

Lichtehberger, E. O., & Kaufman, A. S. (2007). The assessment of preschool children with the Kaufman assessment battery for children-second edition (KABC-II). In B. Bracken & R. Nagle (Eds.), *Psychoeducational assessment of preschool children* (pp. 297–323). Lawrence Erlbaum Associates, Publishers.

Lin, L., Tu, Y., Yu, W., Ho, M., & Wu, P. (2020). Investigation of fine motor performance in children younger than 36-month-old using PDMS-2 and Bayley-III. *European Journal of Developmental Psychology, 17*(5), 746–760. https://doi.org/10.1080/17405629.2020.1732917

Mailend, M. L., Maas, E., Beeson, P. M., Story, B. H., & Forster, K. I. (2020). Speech motor planning in the context of phonetically similar words: Evidence from apraxia of speech and aphasia.

Manfra, L., Squires, C., Dinehart, L. H. B., Bleiker, C., Hartman, S. C., & Winsler, A. (2017). Preschool writing and premathematics predict grade 3 achievement for low-income, ethnically diverse children. *The Journal of Educational Research, 110*(5), 528–537. https://doi.org/10.1080/00220671.2016.1145095

McCrae, J. S., & Brown, S. M. (2018). Systematic review of social-emotional screening instruments for young children in child welfare. *Research on Social Work Practice, 28*(7), 767–788. https://doi.org/10.1177/1049731516686691

McDermott, P. A., Rikoon, S. H., & Fantuzzo, J. W. (2014). Tracing children's approaches to learning through Head Start, kindergarten, and first grade: Different pathways to different outcomes. *Journal of Educational Psychology, 106,* 200–213. https://doi.org/10.1037/a0033547

Michel, G. F., Campbell, J. M., Marcinowski, E. C., Nelson, E. L., & Babik, I. (2016). Infant hand preference and the development of cognitive abilities. *Frontiers in Psychology, 7,* 410. https://doi.org/10.3389/fpsyg.2016.00410

Milne, S., Campbell, L., & Cottier, C. (2020). Accurate assessment of functional abilities in pre-schoolers for diagnostic and funding purposes: A comparison of the Vineland-3 and the PEDI-CAT. *Australian Occupational Therapy Journal, 67*(1), 31–38. https://doi.org/10.1111/1440-1630.12619

Miquelote, A. F., Santos, D. C. C., Caçola, P. M., Montebelo, M. I. L., & Gabbard, C. (2012). Effect of the home environment on motor and cognitive behavior of infants. *Infant Behavior and Development, 35*(3), 329–334. https://doi.org/10.1016/j.infbeh.2012.02.002

Netelenbos, N., Gibb, R. L., Li, F., & Gonzalez, C. L. R. (2018). Articulation speaks to executive function: An investigation in 4-to 6-year-olds. *Frontiers in Psychology, 9*(172). 10.3389/fpsyg.2018.00172

Newborg, J. (2020a). *Battelle developmental inventory* (3rd ed.). Riverside Assessments, LLC.

Newborg, J. (2020b). *Battelle early academic survey.* Riverside Assessments, LLC.

Norbury, C. F. (2013). Practitioner review: Social (pragmatic) communication disorder conceptualization, evidence and clinical implications. *Journal of Child Psychology and Psychiatry, 55,* 204–216. https://doi.org/10.1111/jcpp.12154

Oliver, B. M., & Berger, C. T. (2020). Indiana social-emotional learning competencies: A neurodevelopmental, culturally responsive framework. *Professional School Counseling, 23*(1), 1–10. https://doi.org/10.1177/21/56759X20904486

O'Neil, D. (2009). *Language use inventory.* Knowledge in Development.

Panter, J. E., & Bracken, B. A. (2009). Validity of the Bracken school readiness assessment for predicting first grade readiness. *Psychology in the Schools, 46,* 397–409. https://doi.org/10.1002/pits.20385

Parham, L. D., Ecker, C. L., Kuhaneck, H., Henry, D. A., & Glennon, T. J. (2021). *Sensory processing measure* (2nd ed.). Western Psychological Service.

Reisinger, D. L., Hines, E., Raches, C., Tang, Q., James, C., & Keehn, R. M. (2022). Provider and caregiver satisfaction with telehealth evaluation of autism spectrum disorder in young children during the COVID-19 pandemic. *Journal of Autism and Developmental Disorders, 52,* 5099–5113. https://doi.org/10.1007/s10803-021-04905-0

Reynolds, C. R., & Kamphaus, R. W. (1992). *Manual for the BASC: Behavior assessment system for children.* American Guidance Service.

Reynolds, C. R., & Kamphaus, R. W. (2015). *Behavior assessment system for children—Third edition (BASC-3).* Pearson.

Romano, E., Babchishin, L., Pagani, L. S., & Kohen, D. (2010). School readiness and later achievement: Replication and extension using a nationwide Canadian survey. *Developmental Psychology, 5,* 995–1007. https://doi.org/10.1037/a0018880

Salami, S., Bandeira, P. F. R., Gomes, C. M. A., & Dehkordi, P. S. (2022). The test of gross motor development—Third Edition: A bifactor model, dimensionality, and measurement invariance. *Journal of Motor Learning and Development, 10,* 116–131. https://doi.org/10.1123/jmld.2020-0069

Sanchez, K., Spittle, A. J., Boyce, J. O., Leembruggen, L., Mantelos, A., Mills, S., Mitchell, N., Neil, E., St John, M., Treloar, J., & Morgan, A. T. (2020). Conversational language in 3-year-old children born very preterm and at term. *Journal of Speech, Language, and Hearing Research, 63.* https://doi.org/10.1044/2019_JSLHR-19-00153

Sansavini, A., Favilla, M. E., Guasti, M. T., Marini, A., Millepiedi, S., Di Martino, M. V., Vecchi, S., Battajon, N., Bertolo, L., Capirci, O., Carretti, B., Colatei, M. P., Frioni, C., Marotta, L., Massa, S., Michelazzo, L., Pecini, C., Piazzalunga, S., Pieretti, M., . . . Lorusso, M. L. (2021). Developmental language disorder: Early predictors, age for the diagnosis, and diagnostic tools. A scoping review. *Brain Sciences, 11,* 654–692. https://doi.org/10.3390/brainsci11050654

Santos, E. M. M. D., Constantino, B., Rocha, M. M. D., & Mastroeni, M. F. (2020). Predictors of low perceptual-motor skills in children at 4-5 years of age. *Revista Brasileira de Saude Materno Infantil, 20*(3), 759–767. https://doi.org/10.1590/1806-93042020000300006

Saulnier, C. A., & Klaiman, C. (2022). Assessment of adaptive behavior in autism spectrum disorder. *Psychology in the Schools, 59*(7), 1419–1429. https://doi.org/10.1002/pits.22690

Saulnier, C. A., & Ventola, P. E. (2012). *Essentials of autism spectrum disorders evaluation and assessment.* Wiley.

Schneider, W. J., & McGrew, K. S. (2018). The Cattell-Horn-Carroll theory of cognitive abilities. In D. P. Flanagan & E. M. McDonough (Eds.), *Contemporary intellectual assessment: Theories, tests, and issues* (4th ed., pp. 73–163). The Guilford Press.

Schrank, F. A., McGrew, K. S., & Mather, N. (2015). *Woodcock-Johnson IV tests of early cognitive and academic development.* Houghton Mifflin Harcourt.

Shurman, J., & Leone, D. (2023). Standardized versus naturalized: An evaluation of child morphological and syntactic assessments. *International Journal of Undergraduate Research and Creative Activities, 7,* 1–14. https://doi.org/10.7710/2168-0620.1046

Sotelo-Dynega, M., & Dixon, S. G. (2014). Cognitive assessment practices: A survey of school psychologists. *Psychology in the Schools, 51,* 1031–1045. https://doi.org/10.1002/pits.21802

Sparrow, S. S., Cicchetti, D. V., & Saulnier, C. A. (2016). *Vineland adaptive behavior scales and manual* (3rd ed.). Pearson.

Squires, J., Bricker, D., & Twombly, E. (2015). *Ages and stages questionnaires, social-emotional* (2nd ed.). Brookes Publishing Co.

Taverna, L., Tremolada, M., Bonichini, S., Intra, F. S., & Brighi, A. (2021). Assessing children's gross-motor development: Parent and teacher agreement implication for school and wellbeing. *Journal of Physical Education & Sport, 21,* 560–566.

Thurman, A. J., Bullard, L., Kelly, L., Wong, C., Nguyen, V., Esbensen, A. J., Bekins, J., Schworer, E. K., Fidler, D. J., Daunhauer, L. A., Mervis, C. B., Pitts, C. H., Becerra, A. M., & Abbeduto, L. (2022). Defining expressive language benchmarks for children with down syndrome. *Brain Sciences, 12*(743). https://doi.org/10.3390/brainsci12060743

Tiwari, M., & Tiwari, M. (2012). Voice- How humans communicate? *Journal of National Science, Biology and Medicine, 3*(1), 3–11. https://doi.org/10.4103/0976-9668.95933

U.S. Department of Education. (2020). *OSEP fast facts: Children 3 through 5 served under part B, section 619 of the IDEA*. Individuals with Disabilities Education Act. Retrieved August 7, 2023 from https://sites.ed.gov/idea/osep-fast-facts-children-3-5-20.

Ulrich, D. A. (2019). *Test of gross motor development- Third edition (TGMD-3)*. Pro-Ed.

Ulrich, D. A. (1985). *Test of gross motor development*. Pro-Ed.

Ulrich, D. A. (2000). *The test of gross motor development* (2nd ed.). Pro-Ed.

Van Hartinsveldt, M. J., Cup, E. H. C., Hendricks, J. C. M., de Vries, L., de Groot, I. J. M., & Nijhuis-van der Sanden, M. W. G. (2015). Predictive validity of kindergarten assessments on handwriting readiness. *Research in Developmental Disabilities, 36*, 114–124.

Veiskarami, P., Roozbahani, M., Saedi, S., & Ghadampour, E. (2021). Comparing fine and gross motor development in normal hearing children, rehabilitated, and non-rehabilitated hearing-impaired children. *Auditory & Vestibular Research, 31*(3), 208–217. https://doi.org/10.18502/avr.v31i3.9871

Wahlstrom, D., Raiford, S. E., Breaux, K. C., Zhu, J., & Weiss, L. G. (2018). The wechsler preschool and primary scale of intelligence—fourth edition, wechsler intelligence sale for children—fifth edition, and wechsler individual achievement test—third edition. In D. P. Flanagan & E. M. McDonough (Eds.), *Contemporary intellectual assessment: Theories, tests, and issues* (4th ed., pp. 237–272). The Guilford Press.

Walker, K. C. (1994). Book review: Preschool language scale-3 (PLS-3). *Journal of Psychoeducational Assessment, 12*, 92–97. https://doi.org/10.1177/073428299401200112

Walsh, B., Mettel, K. M., & Smith, A. (2015). Speech motor planning and execution deficits in early childhood stuttering. *Journal of Neurodevelopmental Disorders, 7*(1). https://doi.org/10.1186/s11689-015-9123-8

Wechsler, D. (2002). *Wechsler preschool and primary scale of intelligence* (3rd ed.). Pearson.

Wechsler, D. (2012). *Wechsler preschool and primary scale of intelligence* (4th ed.). Pearson.

Wendling, B. J., Mather, N., LaForte, E. M., McGrew, K. S., & Schrank, F. A. (2015). *Woodcock-Johnson IV tests of early cognitive and academic development*. Houghton Mifflin Harcourt.

Whitcomb, S. A., & Kemp, J. M. (2020). Behavior and socio-emotional skills assessment of preschool children. In V. C. Alfonso, B. B. Bracken, & R. J. Nagle (Eds.), *Psychoeducational assessment of preschool children* (5th ed., pp. 181–203). Routledge.

Wiig, E.H., Secord, W. A., & Semel, E. (2020). Clinical evaluation of language fundamentals preschool–3.Pearson Education.

Wiig, E. H., Secord, W., & Semel, E. (1992). *Clinical evaluation of language fundamentals—preschool*. Psychological Corporation.

Yesnazar, A., Japbarov, A., Zhorabekova, A., Kabylbekova, Z., Nuralieva, A., & Elmira, U. (2021). Elementary school children's speech skills in interdisciplinary ICT communication. *World Journal on Educational Technology: Current Issues, 13*(1), 147–159.

Zevenbergen, A. A., & Ryan, M. M. (2010). Gender differences in the relationship between attention problems and expressive language and emerging academic skills in preschool-aged children. *Early Child Development and Care, 180*, 1337–1348. https://doi.org/10.1080/03004430903059292

Zimmerman, I. L., Steiner, V. G., & Evatt, R. L. (1969). *Preschool Language Scale*. Merrill.

Zimmerman, I. L., Steiner, V. G., & Pond, R. E. (1979). *Preschool language scale*, Revised edition. Merrill.

Zimmerman, I. L., Steiner, V. G., & Pond, R. E. (1992). *Preschool language scale–3*. The Psychological Corporation.

Zimmerman, I. L., Steiner, V. G., & Pond, R. E. (2002). *Preschool language scale* (4th ed.). The Psychological Corporation.

Zimmerman, I. L., Steinerm, V. G., & Pond, R. E. (2011). *Preschool language scale* (5th ed.). Pearson.

Five

ASSESSMENT OF YOUNG CHILDREN WITH LOW INCIDENCE DEVELOPMENTAL AND MEDICAL DISORDERS

Carly G. McDonald, MA, Courtney M., Larsen, MA, & Brittany A. Dale, PhD, HSPP

As introduced earlier in this volume, the passage of the Education of All Handicapped Children Act (Public Law 94-142; United States Congress, 1975) in 1975 marked a historical moment in the education of children with disabilities by ensuring that they were entitled to receive special education services in the schools. Prior to 1975, young children with the most significant needs would have been excluded from the educational system. It took even longer for federal laws to be amended to ensure infants and toddlers with diagnosed medical conditions or who were exhibiting developmental delays could have access to early intervention services. It was not until 1986 that federal laws were amended to provide services for infants, toddlers, and preschoolers who have significant needs (Markelz & Batement, 2021).

Young children with the most significant needs often fall under the broad category of low incidence disabilities, indicating that these disabilities and medical disorders have low prevalence rates. According to the Individuals with Disabilities Education Act (IDEA, 2004), this category includes those with visual and hearing impairments, co-occurring visual and hearing impairment, significant cognitive impairment, and any impairment for which a small number of highly skilled personnel are needed for interventions. These young children often have unique medical and educational needs; thus, examiners should be aware of how these unique needs may affect developmental and educational evaluations. This chapter discusses several low incidence disabilities (e.g., those with genetic disorders, intellectual disabilities, traumatic brain injury, autism, and deafblindness)

Essentials of Assessing Infants, Toddlers, and Preschoolers, First Edition.
Brittany A. Dale, Joseph R. Engler, and Vincent C. Alfonso.
© 2025 John Wiley & Sons, Inc. Published 2025 by John Wiley & Sons, Inc.

and provides special considerations that examiners should consider when evaluating those populations. We begin with a discussion of various genetic conditions and the unique developmental qualities that are characteristic of young children with these conditions. We then describe the various assessment considerations for young children suspected of intellectual disability, a common comorbidity of many of the genetic conditions included in this chapter. Assessment considerations for young children who have experienced a traumatic brain injury, and those in the low incidence categories of deafblindness and deaf and hard of hearing are also included. Although no longer considered low-incidence, autism spectrum disorder is included here because of the specialized training recommended for examiners assessing ASD (Corona et al., 2021; Margiano et al., 2023). We end by discussing medical disorders that may uniquely impact the assessment of young children.

CAUTION 5.1

Although this chapter presents information on many low incidence disabilities, this is not an exhaustive list of all possible conditions with which young children may present.

GENETIC DISORDERS

It is important for examiners to understand the characteristics of common genetic disorders prior to assessing young children with developmental delays. Genetic disorders result from mutations in the genetic code or when an individual has the incorrect amount of genetic material (Cleveland Clinic, 2021a). Some genetic disorders include Down Syndrome, Fragile-X, Turner's Syndrome, Angelman Syndrome, and Williams Syndrome. These disorders account for approximately 40% of individuals diagnosed with global developmental delay and intellectual disability (Miclea et al., 2015). Furthermore, children may be born with chromosomal abnormalities that are not linked to known or discovered genetic disorders. These children may have atypical physical symptoms, predispositions to medical conditions, and unique patterns of developmental delays (Miclea et al., 2015).

Many genetic disorders place infants, toddlers, and preschoolers at higher risk for physical, mental, and behavioral challenges. Therefore, examiners must be familiar with related health concerns prior to assessing the child. For instance, an examiner should ensure that hearing and vision have been screened. This can be done by establishing a comprehensive developmental history from the parent's report. In addition, all infants receive a hearing test at birth, and psychologists and other professionals (e.g., school nurses and teachers) should follow up with parents to learn if more recent testing has been completed. Hearing and vision screening can also occur at school and during a multidisciplinary team evaluation.

Children from low incidence populations may also benefit from the creation of an Individualized Health Plan (IHP). IHPs are essential for students whose medical conditions may negatively impact their ability to access their education (National Association of School Nurses, 2020). They are separate from an Individualized Education Program (IEP) and are not contingent upon the child qualifying for an IEP or a Section 504 plan. Examiners and other school staff (i.e., principals, general and special educators, speech language pathologists, etc.) will likely collaborate with the school medical staff to provide relevant information on the child's performance when considering an IHP. Specifically, school nurses will coordinate with the young child's family, the school, and external community-based health care services to ensure the young child's health care needs are met (Kruzliakova et al., 2021). The IHP outlines all the medical services a child would need throughout their school day to support school performance and optimize school attendance. It outlines not only the medical services that are needed, but also any mental health services that are necessary. The IHP will aid in the continuity of care throughout the young child's day by allowing everyone to be on the same page with the child's medical needs. Comprehensive evaluation of the young child's developmental skills can inform the team of the child's functioning when developing these plans.

The following sections provide an overview of and relevant research for common genetic disorders that examiners may encounter. These sections should not be considered exhaustive of all potential genetic disorders with which infants, toddlers, and preschoolers could be diagnosed. We include a description of each condition, prevalence, associated developmental delays, unique needs, and diagnostic considerations of common genetic disorders.

Fragile-X Syndrome

Fragile-X Syndrome (FXS), also known as Martin–Bell Syndrome, is a genetic disorder that results from changes in the gene *FMR1* (Berry-Kravis et al., 2011). There are different forms of *FMR1* mutations that FXS can result from, all of which take place on the X-chromosome. FXS is diagnosed with a blood test; however, young children may be suspected of FXS if they present with the common physical features of the disorder (see Rapid Reference 5.1). It is the most common form of inherited intellectual disabilities and developmental delay for individuals (Stone et al., 2017). Due to the sex-gene nature of the disorder, males are more severely impacted by FXS than females (Bartholomay et al., 2019; Keysor & Mazzocco, 2002). For example, approximately 64% of females and 96% of males are diagnosed with co-occurring developmental delay or intellectual disability (Bailey et al., 2008). Females with FXS have varying cognitive abilities ranging from a moderate intellectual disability to average or above intellectual functioning (De Vries et al., 1996; Hagerman et al., 1992; Tsiouris & Brown, 2004), whereas males with FXS are more likely to have severe intellectual disabilities (Backes et al., 2000). Furthermore, research shows females with FXS have specific difficulties with mathematics (Lachiewicz et al., 2006).

The average age of an FXS diagnosis is around 35 months for males and 42 months for females (Bailey et al., 2009); however, studies suggest that with screening tools (e.g., Battelle Developmental Inventory Screening Test-2, Newborg, J. 2005; Early Language Milestone Scale-2, Coplan, 1993), children can be diagnosed with FXS as young as 9 months old (Mirrett et al., 2004). Furthermore, research shows parents express developmental concerns about their children before the child's first birthday, with the first concerns being related to motor delays (Zhang et al., 2017). Toddlers with FXS have delayed developmental milestones, such as challenges with coordination, speech, and social skills (Abbeduto & Murphy, 2004; Friefeld & Macgregor, 1994). Additionally, 10–20% of people with FXS have epilepsy (Berry-Kravis, 2002), and many children with FXS have difficulty falling asleep and/or staying asleep (Kronk et al., 2009, 2010).

Children with FXS may be diagnosed with comorbid conditions, such as autism spectrum disorder (Stone et al., 2017). Research suggests 27%–81% of males and approximately 21% of females with FXS also meet the criteria for autism; thus, understanding the nature of the overlap is important for the treatment planning of FXS (Hall et al., 2008; Sterling, 2018). Specifically, poor eye contact (Hall et al., 2009), hand flapping (Hagerman, 1999), and speech difficulties such as preservative and noncontingent speech are common across conditions (Diez-Itza et al., 2022; Martin et al., 2012). While sharing commonalities, it is important to note differences between the presentation of ASD in children with FXS compared to idiopathic autism (i.e., when cause is unknown; Moss & Howlin, 2009). Specifically, individuals with FXS are more likely to have social withdrawal associated with social anxiety and shyness (Moss & Howlin, 2009). Additionally, they have different developmental trajectories and preserved emotional sensitivity (Hatton et al., 2006; Shaw & Porter, 2013). Lastly, males with FXS commonly engage in self-injurious behaviors such as biting of hands and fingers (Symons et al., 2003, 2010).

Rapid Reference 5.1 Common Physical Features of Children with FXS

- Elongated face
- Larger head circumference
- Large ears
- Prominent jaw
- Males have abnormally large testes

Source: Adapted from Hagerman (2002).

Down Syndrome

Down Syndrome (DS), also referred to as Trisomy 21, is a genetic disorder that most commonly is a result of an additional copy of chromosome 21; however, 3% of children with DS are diagnosed with Translocation Down Syndrome, which results from genetic material from chromosome 21 attached or translocated to a different chromosome (Center for Disease Control [CDC], 2021). Furthermore, 2% of children with DS have some cells with three copies of chromosome 21, and other cells with the typical number which is called Mosaic Down Syndrome (CDC, 2021; Shin et al., 2010). One in every 700 babies is diagnosed with DS (Mai et al., 2019). Routine prenatal screenings, including blood testing and ultrasounds, typically identify DS during pregnancy.

Children with DS have physical, cognitive, and motor development that differs from typically developing children. For example, individuals with DS have low muscle tone, flattened faces, shorter height, and a shorter neck (CDC, 2021). Some individuals with DS have major birth defects such as hearing problems (75%), eye disease (60%), and heart defects

(50%; Bull et al., 2011). Individuals with DS also have varying cognitive profiles (Onnivello et al., 2022). For example, some individuals display relative strengths in visual-spatial skills and implicit memory but have relative weaknesses with language and verbal memory (Grieco et al., 2015; Jarrold et al. 2008). Deficits in expressive language, syntactic processing, and delayed speech processing skills are also noted (Patterson, 2007). Thus, school staff should design interventions and supports for young children with DS based on their unique cognitive and behavioral profile, which can only be determined through accurate assessment. Individuals with DS typically have poor fine and gross motor skills (CDC, 2021). Motor development should be targeted with early intervention as it is shown to be associated with cognitive development for infants with DS (Diedrichsen et al., 2010; Malak et al., 2013).

Children with DS are commonly included in the standardization samples of developmental and early childhood norm-referenced measures. Infants and toddlers 1 month to 42 months of age with DS can be assessed across developmental domains (i.e., cognitive, language, motor, social-emotional, and adaptive) using the Bayley Scales of Infant and Toddler Development, Fourth Edition (Bayley-4; Bayley & Aylward, 2019) or the Battelle Developmental Inventory, 3rd Edition (BDI-3; Newborg, 2020). Both comprehensive developmental assessments included children with DS in the standardization samples, making them appropriate assessment tools for this population.

> **DON'T FORGET 5.1**
>
> Many standardized developmental and intellectual measures included children with DS in the standardization sample, making them appropriate to use with this population.

Turner Syndrome

Turner Syndrome (TS) is a sex-based chromosomal abnormality that affects approximately one in every 2,500 females (Cleveland Clinic, 2021b). TS is diagnosed when genetic testing reveals an intact X chromosome with a missing second X chromosome or a partially altered second X chromosome; therefore, only females are affected. Age of diagnosis varies depending on the symptoms presented. Approximately one-third are diagnosed as a newborn due to puffy hands and feet or redundant nuchal skin; another one-third are diagnosed mid-childhood due to short stature; and the remainder are diagnosed later in life related to failure to enter puberty and/or difficulty achieving pregnancy (Sybert & McCauley, 2004). Examiners and educators should be aware of the potential medical complications that may affect an infant or toddler with TS. Specifically, individuals with TS are more likely to have congenital heart defects and kidney problems (Lippe et al., 1988; Sybert, 1998). Individualized Family Service Plan (IFSP) and IEP teams should be aware of an infant's or toddler's medical complications when planning assessment and intervention recommendations. See Rapid Reference 5.2 for a list of common physical characteristics with TS.

Many females with TS have typical cognitive functioning (Sybert & McCauley, 2004). However, 10% of individuals with TS have developmental delays and an intellectual disability (Gravholt et al., 2017). Specifically, developmental delays may occur in fine motor, gross motor, and language skills (Robinson et al., 1990). Additionally, children with TS often have a learning disability, affecting their nonverbal abilities such as visuospatial and executive skills, visual working memory, and mathematics (Mazzocco, 2006; Rourke, 1995).

≋ Rapid Reference 5.2 Physical Features of Children with Turner Syndrome

Physical Features

- Short stature
- Premature ovarian failure
- "Webbed" neck
- Low hairline at the back of the neck
- Swelling of the hands and feet
- Skeletal abnormalities

Note: Not all these symptoms may be present. For more information.
Source: Adapted from https://rarediseases.info.nih.gov/diseases/7831/turner-syndrome.

Angelman Syndrome

Angelman Syndrome (AS) is a genetic disorder that affects approximately 1 in 15,000 children (Margolis et al., 2015). Children with AS have developmental delays (e.g., speech, motor, and cognitive) which become noticeable around 6 months of age (Williams et al., 2010). However, children with AS often initially receive a misdiagnosis or undergo extensive diagnostic testing, delaying the time of diagnosis to 21–46 months (Mertz et al., 2013). Infants and toddlers with AS are at a higher risk for seizures, with 80% experiencing seizures (Clayton-Smith & Laan, 2003; Margolis et al., 2015). The onset of seizures varies but commonly occurs around 18–24 months of age. Many young children with AS also experience sleep problems, such as reduced sleep time, night awakening, and night terrors (Pelc et al., 2008). Additionally, most children with AS have motor impairments ranging from the inability to walk to fine motor deficits (Wheeler et al., 2017). Specifically, jerky movements are common in the first months of life and motor delays (e.g., difficulty crawling and sitting up unsupported) may become apparent at approximately 9 months of age (Clayton-Smith & Pembrey, 1992).

Children with AS typically have severe to profound intellectual disabilities (Andersen et al., 2001; Clayton-Smith & Laan, 2003), which may present challenges during the assessment process. Specifically, children with AS display significant expressive language delays, with many children being nonverbal (see Rapid Reference 5.3; Clayton-Smith & Pembrey, 1992). Therefore, examiners may need to alter their typical evaluation techniques by choosing developmentally appropriate measures rather than measures that account for the child's chronological age (Andersen et al., 2001). For example, examiners may need to utilize the tasks from developmental measures intended for use with infants and toddlers when assessing a preschool-aged child with AS, even if the child is too old based on the standardized administration procedures. Rather than relying on standard interpretation, examiners should provide a narrative interpretation of development including the child's current skills as obtained on the measure. For a toddler, they may need to alter start points to account for a toddler's developmental delays and make sure they are familiar with items typically administered to infants.

CAUTION 5.2

Examiners may not be able to rely on standardized interpretation of assessments for children with AS. Narrative descriptions of the infant, toddler, or preschool child's skills may be more informative to the intervention team.

Research suggests individuals with AS have a relative weakness in motor skills and a relative strength in socialization skills (Andersen et al., 2001). Despite stronger socialization skills compared to other skills, they may exhibit inappropriate laughter provoked from the smallest stimulus (Clayton-Smith & Laan, 2003) and act inappropriately in social situations. Therefore, it is important to assess their adaptive skills to target and create a specific goal in the social skills domain.

≡ *Rapid Reference 5.3 Physical Features and Developmental Delays Associated with Children with Angelman Syndrome*

Physical Features	Developmental Delays
• Prominent chin • Deep-set eyes • Wide mouth • Protruding tongue • Smaller head • Frequent drooling	• Severe expressive language difficulty, including lack of speech and/ or only acquiring a few words • Motor dysfunction • Delayed crawling (18–24 months) and walking (4 years)

Sources: Clayton-Smith and Laan (2003) and Margolis et al. (20165).

Williams Syndrome

Williams Syndrome (WS) is a rare genetic disorder caused by the deletion of 26 continuous genes on chromosome 7 q11.23 (Morris, 2010). Prevalence estimates range from approximately 1 in 7,500 to 1 in 20,000 children (Mervis et al., 2003; Strømme et al., 2002). Young children with WS commonly exhibit developmental delays, physical abnormalities, and unique personality characteristics. See Rapid Reference 5.4 for examples of these features. Additionally, many have cardiovascular problems, including hypertension and supravalvar aortic stenosis (a narrowing of blood vessels in the heart that develops before birth; Mervis & Morris, 2007; Morris, 2010). Infants with WS experience chronic ear infections, constipation, feeding difficulties, hypotonia, and lax joints. Due to feeding and other physical difficulties, these infants may be categorized as failure to thrive. Ninety-five percent of young children with WS experience hyperacusis, which "is an oversensitivity or excessive perception of normal environmental sounds" (p. 390, Gothelf et al., 2006). Examiners should be aware of these unique features and consult with an audiologist to assess any measured hearing differences and manage the child's sensitivity to noise.

Similar to many other genetic disorders reviewed in this chapter, individuals with WS often have intellectual disabilities with variable peaks and valleys across their cognitive profiles (Pezzini et al., 1999). They display relative strengths in verbal short-term memory and language and weaknesses in visuospatial construction (Mervis & Morris, 2007). Despite the higher numbers with mild intellectual disabilities, some individuals with WS have average cognitive functioning (Mervis & Morris, 2007). Other comorbidities include attention deficit hyperactivity disorder (ADHD) and oppositional defiant disorder (Leyfer et al., 2006). Specifically, people with WS are likely to have increased oppositional behaviors, impaired working memory, and difficulty planning (Rhodes et al., 2011).

WS is often characterized by reduced social inhibition, which makes these children appear overly friendly and often show "marked friendliness to adults including strangers" (p.142, Pezzini et al., 1999). Consequently, children with WS may be more vulnerable to exploitation in social situations and may require targeted social skills interventions.

Rapid Reference 5.4 Physical Features and Developmental Delays Associated with Children with Williams Syndrome

Physical Features	Developmental Delays
• Broad forehead	• Delayed onset of speech
• Short nose	• Difficulty with pragmatics in speech
• Wide mouth	
• Small jaw	• Impaired memory
• Large ear lobes	• Slow sensorimotor development
• Abnormal alignment of the eyes	
• Poor weight gain early in life	
• Hoarse voice	

Sources: Mervis and Morris (2007), Mervis and Velleman (2011), Pezzini et al. (1999), and Sampaio et al. (2008).

GENETIC DISORDERS: IMPLICATIONS FOR ASSESSMENT

As noted above, intellectual disabilities often accompany several of the genetic disorders described. Examiners must take care in selecting appropriate cognitive abilities measures, especially for the preschool population where measures of intelligence often do not have appropriate floors. The following section discusses more implications for the assessment of intellectual disabilities. Additionally, although research suggests that young children with genetic disorders may exhibit cognitive profiles specific to the disorder, examiners must provide the most appropriate intervention recommendations based on the individual's unique strengths and weaknesses.

Assessment for differential diagnosis of other neurodevelopmental disorders is also imperative when conducting an evaluation for a young child with a known genetic disorder. For instance, young boys with FXS may present with symptoms of ADHD, as it is a common comorbid disorder (Sullivan et al., 2006). During an assessment, the examiner should note any hyperactive or inattentive behaviors observed from the child and take frequent breaks. Standardized, norm-referenced tests may need to be broken down into smaller portions to avoid fatigue. Although these are good strategies to utilize with any young child, extra accommodations may be needed with special populations.

To ensure the most valid interpretation, best practices suggest examiners should consider using tests that include the genetic disorder in the standardization sample for their assessment. For instance, the Bayley-4 included children with DS in the normative sample, which supports its use for infants and toddlers with DS (Bayley & Aylward, 2019).

Whenever possible, examiners should also consider using an interdisciplinary assessment approach when assessing genetic disorders as many children with genetic disorders have comorbid health conditions (see Chapter 6, this volume, for a further discussion on interdisciplinary assessment). Research shows that working in collaboration within interdisciplinary teams is more effective for treatment than working in isolation (Arora et al., 2019; Kerins, 2018). In a preschool setting, school psychologists could collaborate with the school nurse, registered dietitian nutritionist, mental health counselors, and teachers to gain a full picture of the child's developmental and medical needs to inform the best treatment for the child (McIntosh et al., 2021). Additionally, depending on the child's developmental delays related to motor and sensory concerns, an occupational and/or physical therapist will aid in the direct assessment in those areas. Lastly, examiners should consider using a multimodal assessment approach to gain a fuller picture of the child's abilities and current functioning. Chapter 6 of this volume provides more information on multidisciplinary and interdisciplinary evaluations.

INTELLECTUAL DISABILITY

Many of the genetic disorders discussed in the previous section of this chapter have Intellectual Developmental Disorder (IDD; also referred to as Intellectual Disability) as a clinical feature. Approximately 3% of the population is estimated to have an IDD (Patel et al., 2020). The *Diagnostic and Statistical Manual of Mental Disorders – Fifth Edition, Text Revision* (DSM-5-TR; American Psychiatric Association [APA], 2022) defines an IDD as deficits in intellectual and adaptive functioning that are approximately two or more standard deviations below the mean on standardized assessment. Onset occurs during the developmental period, making assessment of young children vital to establishing a history of underdeveloped skills. The standard error of measurement should be considered (e.g., standard scores in the 65–75 range for tests with a Mean = 100 and Standard Deviation = 15) when determining if a child qualifies for a diagnosis, and the severity (e.g., mild, moderate, severe, and profound) of an individual's impairment should be determined by their level of adaptive functioning within the areas of conceptual, social, and practical skills (APA, 2022).

Furthermore, the severity of the IDD impacts what age-identifiable developmental delays will appear. In general, the more severe the IDD, the earlier the developmental delay will appear. For example, children with severe or profound IDD are more likely to have identifiable delays that prompt testing as early as 2 years old (APA, 2022) or earlier. According to the DSM-5-TR, when a child is *under* the age of 5 years and the examiner is not confident in standardized testing results or the young child is unable to participate in testing, the diagnosis of Global Developmental Delay may be given. The examiner must determine that the child fails to meet several intellectual developmental milestones, which can be done through developmental rating scales, observations, and other developmental tools (i.e., comprehensive developmental measures). A Global Developmental Delay diagnosis, according to the DSM-5-TR, is defined more broadly compared to educational law and could provide the opportunity for the child to receive early intervention services in a clinic setting when medical insurance requires documentation of "medical necessity" for treatment. Infant and toddler cognitive abilities, as described elsewhere in this volume, are commonly assessed through standardized developmental assessments that include a cognitive domain. The Bayley-4 (Bayley & Aylward, 2019) and the BDI-3 (Newborg, 2020) are two measures that can be used to help support a Global Developmental Delay diagnosis as defined by the DSM-5-TR as well as Developmental Delay as defined by IDEA.

The genetic disorders discussed earlier can be the cause of IDD. However, IDD is not always attributed to biological factors (Karam et al., 2016). Nonbiological factors include environmental factors (e.g., teratogens, viruses) or injury (e.g., head trauma or lack of oxygen to the brain). There are varying estimates of how many children have an IDD due to biological or nonbiological causes (Karam et al., 2016; McLaren & Bryson, 1987).

As described in Chapters 2 and 3 of this volume, cognitive tests used to assess toddlers and preschoolers must be evaluated for their quantitative and qualitative (e.g., representation of IDD in the standardization sample, appropriate floors, etc.) properties prior to selection for an evaluation. Tests with suboptimal floors can be problematic when comparing cognitive abilities to adaptive functioning. For example, several cognitive measures have a standard score floor of 40, which is four standard deviations below the mean, while some measures of adaptive behavior have a standard score floor of 20, which is 5 standard deviations below the mean. Selection of tools with appropriate floors is vital for an assessment of IDD. Rapid Reference 5.5 lists several important assessment considerations when evaluating young children for IDD or Global Developmental Delay.

≡ Rapid Reference 5.5 Assessment Considerations for IDD

- Choose test measures with appropriate floors (Bracken, 1987; Bradley-Johnson, 2001)
- Infant and toddler developmental measures have better floor properties for older toddlers since the measure includes items designed for the youngest of children. Examiners may need to begin at a start point for a younger child if necessary.

(continued)

> ### ≋ *Rapid Reference 5.5*
>
> *(continued)*
>
> - Examiners might consider using assessments that are intended for younger children and provide a qualitative interpretation. For example, a school psychologist might consider using some of the Bayley-4 tasks with a 4-year-old child to provide recommendations for interventions based on their qualitative performance.
> - Adaptive measures should be given more weight (Boat et al., 2015).
> - When individualized standardized assessment is inappropriate for the young child, parent report rating scales may be necessary to determine the current level of functioning. Standard scores many be obtained from these rating scales; however, examiners should interpret these as estimates of cognitive functioning.

TRAUMATIC BRAIN INJURIES

Traumatic brain injuries (TBI) result from injury (e.g., falls, abuse, and motor vehicle accidents) to the scalp, skull, and/or brain (Araki et al., 2017). TBIs can occur without apparent bleeding or physical markings and can lead to physical disabilities, intellectual disabilities, and/or death (Araki et al., 2017). Every year, over 139,000 children under the age of 5 years end up in the emergency room from a fall-related injury and are diagnosed with a TBI (Haarbauer-Krupa et al., 2019). Sadly, many infants are hospitalized for abusive head trauma, such as shaken baby syndrome, at a rate of 35 cases per 100,000 infants (Joyce et al., 2022). Every year, approximately 1.5 in 100,000 children have TBI-related deaths (Spencer & Hedegaard, 2020). Research indicates that age at the time of the injury is a large predictor of child outcomes, with younger children fairing worse (Anderson et al., 2004; Kriel et al., 1989; Lange-Cosack et al., 1979). Specifically, children under the age of 6 years have worse cognitive and motor outcomes compared to children older than 6 years (Kriel et al., 1989).

TBI recovery for young children (2 years to 6 years 11 months old) depends on the severity of the injury (Anderson et al., 2004). Anderson and colleagues summarized developmental recovery well, and examiners should consult their research for more specific information on TBI outcomes for young children. In summary, they found that for children who had typical development prior to injury, those who had severe TBI injuries displayed a significant decline in cognitive and language functioning when tested at 3, 12, and 30 months post injury, whereas children with mild and moderate TBI injuries did not have a significant decline in cognitive and language functioning. Language recovery for expressive language occurred across all TBI groups, but not for receptive language. Memory recovery occurred for the mild and moderate TBI groups; however, the severe TBI group had reduced memory performance. Children in the severe TBI group performed the poorest across all measures 30 months post injury. Similarly, research using a toddler population indicated that toddlers with severe TBIs do not have significant improvements in cognitive, motor, and language scores 6 months post injury (Ewing-Cobbs et al., 1997).

The above research suggests that examiners should have a solid understanding of potential TBI recovery outcomes for young children depending on the severity and timing of the injury. Prior to developing an assessment plan, examiners must gather a thorough developmental history of the young child's functioning prior to the accident or injury, medical records indicating the level of severity, timeline of the child's physical recovery, and current functional level. Interprofessional collaboration may be necessary for a complete understanding of the young child's medical history; therefore, examiners should obtain the proper mutual exchange of information releases to facilitate this collaboration. Results of testing should be used by the child's intervention team to develop an appropriate treatment plan in whatever setting (e.g., home, school, or clinic) the infant, toddler, or preschool child will receive services.

Since TBI is one of the 13 federally defined special education categories for preschool children (see Rapid Reference 1.2 in Chapter 1 of this volume for a list of IDEA special education categories), examiners should help educate parents on the benefits of an IEP when deficits are identified through assessment. Early interventionists and early childhood special education teachers must be aware of the potential outcomes as some children may struggle to return to their baseline functioning after a TBI, especially those who experienced a severe TBI. Ongoing assessment of young children with TBI is essential to maintain appropriate intervention goals and determine the extent of cognitive decline.

DON'T FORGET 5.2

Severity of injury and age of injury for young children with TBI affect recovery outcomes.

DEAFBLINDNESS

Deafblindness is a rare condition that involves a combination of hearing and vision loss. In the United States, there are approximately 2,000 children, ages 0–60 months, who have been identified as deafblind (National Center on Deaf-Blindness [NCDB], 2020). Although deafblindness is considered the smallest disability group under the IDEA, there is much heterogeneity within this population in terms of severity and type of hearing and vision loss (Bruce et al., 2018). For some individuals, deafblindness involves a complete absence of hearing and sight. However, in most cases, these senses are reduced but not missing entirely, with 99% of children with deafblindness having some residual hearing or vision (NCDB, 2020). The etiology of deafblindness is variable, ranging from hereditary syndromes and disorders (e.g., Usher Syndrome and DS) to postnatal causes, such as asphyxia, meningitis, and physical injuries (Miles, 2008). In total, there are over 70 known causes of deafblindness, many of which can result in other disabilities (NCDB, 2020). By one estimate, nearly 90% of children with deafblindness have at least one other disability, including speech/language impairments, physical impairments, and cognitive impairments (NCDB, 2020). As this brief overview illustrates, individuals with deafblindness have diverse characteristics, necessitating highly specialized assessment and programming.

In recent years, the assessment of individuals with hearing or vision loss has become increasingly standardized (Nicholas, 2020). For example, a technical report was published to provide guidance on administering the WPPSI-IV (Wechsler, 2012) to children who are deaf or hard of hearing (Costa et al., 2015). However, individuals with deafblindness are less likely to benefit from these recommendations, as two senses are affected rather than one. The interaction between concurrent sensory deficits (e.g., hearing impairment and visual impairment) is complex, and the effects cannot be measured by simply adding the sensory deficits together (van Dijk et al., 2010). The multiplicative effect of dual sensory impairment is illustrated by van Dijk et al. (2010):

> A person with an average hearing loss of 60 decibels will have difficulties understanding a person speaking to him in a noisy environment. The person will try to compensate for his hearing impairment by watching the speaker's face in order to receive additional information. It can be assumed that this person will be able to receive most of the exchanged information. However, if this person has a vision loss of 70% in addition to hearing loss, it is very likely that the speaker's facial expressions and the shape of his mouth will be difficult to discern. In this instance, the person will miss almost all of the conversation. (p. 177)

As this example illustrates, the appropriate accommodations for an individual with vision loss or hearing loss may be insufficient for an individual with impairments in both. Whereas a deaf or hard of hearing child may benefit from interpretation in sign language, this accommodation may be inaccessible to a child with deafblindness. Therefore, the assessment of a child with deafblindness requires careful consideration of their abilities. Evaluations of young children with deafblindness should be completed by specialists who have experience working with this disability category as well as experience with young children. As a low incidence disability, it is likely that families will struggle to find assessment specialists in outpatient clinics. School districts will likely have access to specialists within the state, but they might require extended deadlines for evaluations if these specialists are covering most of the school districts across the state. Similarly, the statewide early intervention programs will likely have specialists that support the entire state or large portions.

Despite the paucity of research on the assessment of children with deafblindness, scholars agree that it is inappropriate to rely solely on standardized assessments. Due to the low incidence of deafblindness, as well as its heterogeneity, children with deafblindness are rarely included as a normative group (Bruce et al., 2018). Furthermore, the results may be invalidated by the accommodations or adaptations needed to administer the assessment to a child with deafblindness (Bruce et al., 2018). When standardized assessments are adapted for use with children with sensory impairments, the scores often underrepresent the child's true abilities (van Dijk et al., 2010). Therefore, a more dynamic approach to assessment is generally recommended. One recommended approach is authentic assessment, which considers the child's abilities, interests, and preferences within the context of their everyday environment (Rowland, 2009). Authentic assessment involves a multidisciplinary team that works together to understand the child's communication skills, motor and sensory abilities, cognitive and social development, and adaptive functioning (Rowland, 2009). In addition, authentic assessment adopts a strengths-based approach that considers the unique attributes of the child, such as their preferences and temperament.

CAUTION 5.3

Individuals with deafblindness are not included in most standardized assessments. Authentic assessment, involving a multidisciplinary team that works together to understand the child's comprehensive functioning, should be utilized.

DEAF AND HARD OF HEARING

The deaf and hard of hearing (DHH) population is a diverse group that includes approximately 100,000 children under the age of 5 years in the United States (U.S. Census Bureau, 2018). The type and severity of hearing loss varies from child to child, which creates a broad array of medical and educational implications. Although *deaf* and *hard of hearing* are grouped together, it is important to note that they are distinct terms. In general, deaf and hard of hearing are differentiated by the degree of hearing loss. Children who are hard of hearing typically have some residual hearing, whereas deafness refers to hearing loss so profound that the child has little to no hearing (World Health Organization, 2021).

Some children are prelingually deaf, meaning that they are born deaf or become deaf before learning to talk. Others experience hearing loss after they have already learned to talk or sometime later in life. Furthermore, hearing loss has many different causes, ranging from genetic to environmental factors. In developed countries, the most common cause of congenital hearing loss is genetics, such as mutations of the genes *GJB2* and *STRC* (Shearer et al., 2023). Although most genetic causes are nonsyndromic (i.e., not connected with other conditions), there are also over 400 syndromes associated with hearing loss. These include Waardenburg Syndrome, Usher Syndrome, and Pendred Syndrome (Shearer et al., 2023). Environmental causes of hearing loss include maternal infections during pregnancy (e.g., rubella) and complications during the perinatal period (e.g., asphyxia at birth).

DON'T FORGET 5.3

Deaf and hard of hearing are differentiated by the degree of hearing loss. Children who are hard of hearing typically have some residual hearing, whereas deafness refers to hearing loss so profound that the child has little to no hearing.

In the United States, early detection of hearing loss has significantly improved over the past 30 years. This is in large part due to legislative mandates requiring universal newborn hearing screenings. By 1992, only two states (Hawaii and Rhode Island) had legislative mandates related to universal newborn hearing screenings; since then, that number has risen to 43 states (Early Hearing Detection and Intervention [EHDI], 2022). Today, many newborns are screened for hearing loss before leaving the hospital, with 98% being screened by 1 month of age (EHDI, 2022).

During these screenings, medical providers use simple tests to see how the brain or inner ear responds to sound. Infants who do not pass the hearing screening undergo further evaluation, usually by 3 months of age (White, 2014).

Early detection is crucial in facilitating early intervention. For infants with diagnosed hearing loss, intervention services should start as early as possible, but no later than 6 months of age (White, 2014). The first few years of life are vital in the acquisition of speech and language skills, and hearing loss may hinder the development of these skills. Research suggests that DHH infants and toddlers should be exposed to language through amplification, American sign language (ASL), or other methods during the critical period, birth through age 5 years (Hall et al., 2017; Lyness et al., 2013). Children who are not exposed to reciprocal language during this time may experience mental health problems, social impairments, and language delays. Early intervention services help children with hearing loss learn how to interact and communicate with others, such as through ASL. Depending on the type and severity of hearing loss, amplification or assistive technology, such as hearing aids or cochlear implants, may be used.

It is important to consider the family's needs when planning assessments to inform interventions for DHH young children. Moreover, examiners should understand the family's stance on assistive technology, whole language, ASL, and other interventions to improve amplification for the child. For instance, families who have embraced the Deaf culture may not be open to suggestions of using cochlear implants. When conducting evaluations for DHH infants and toddlers who communicate through ASL, the examiner should request the presence of an interpreter. Although a family member may be able to interpret for a hearing professional, their role is to be the family member and not the interpreter. Often, hearing psychologists rely on a family member to interpret for their Deaf child, which is not considered best practice in assessment (Dale & Neild, 2020).

In educational settings, the evaluation of preschool DHH children requires a multidisciplinary approach. An IEP team of a preschool child includes a deaf and hard of hearing teacher of record, an audiologist, and potentially a school psychologist who works with Deaf children, in addition to the typical team members. Due to the unique characteristics of DHH students, specialized assessment is required across a variety of domains, including linguistic, social, emotional, physical, and cognitive development.

Furthermore, many DHH individuals have at least one other disability, with estimates ranging from 35 to 50% (Leppo et al., 2014). The high incidence of co-occurring disabilities means that there may be other educational implications. One of the most important aspects of the evaluation is an audiological assessment to understand the nature and degree of the child's hearing. These evaluations are conducted by specialists, such as audiologists, otologists, or otolaryngologists. Audiological evaluations can also provide information about the child's auditory function with amplification and assistive technology. For example, the child may be able to perceive speech normally with a cochlear implant or hearing aids. Another important part of the evaluation process is understanding the child's communication abilities. A speech language pathologist can help assess a child's signed or spoken language abilities.

Evaluating young DHH children poses a unique challenge for school psychologists, who often have limited to no experience working with this population. If there are no specialized school psychologists available to the school district, special considerations must be made. Before beginning their portion of the evaluation, school psychologists should ascertain the child's primary mode of communication. According to the National Association of School Psychologists (NASP), a school psychologist who lacks fluency in the child's primary mode of communication may seek assistance from another qualified professional, such as a sign language interpreter (NASP, 2020). However, the school psychologist must ensure that the interpreter has appropriate training and experience with standardized assessment. The school psychologist should work with the interpreter to ensure that test items are presented as intended and the child's responses are presented back to the examiner verbatim. The school psychologist must also consider that translation from English to ASL is often not a one-for-one translation; therefore, verbal intelligence tests are often not recommended for use and interpretation with Deaf children (Costa et al., 2015).

Examiners are also responsible for selecting instruments that provide a valid representation of the child's abilities. The first step is to consider whether the standardization sample is an appropriate comparison group for the examinee. For example, the WPPSI-IV general normative sample includes children with corrected hearing loss, but not children with uncorrected hearing loss. Many cognitive assessments are heavily dependent upon spoken language for verbal and nonverbal tasks. For many DHH students,

English is a second or unknown language, so they may have had limited access to the content being tested. In fact, DHH students tend to score one standard deviation lower than their hearing peers on measures of verbal intelligence (Whitaker & Thomas-Presswood, 2017). Even on nonverbal subtests, there are significant demands on spoken language, such as in the delivery of instructions. Use of standardized assessments should be considered with care. Although standardized assessments provide valuable information, examiners should proceed with caution when interpreting the results. Undue emphasis on standardized assessments may paint an inaccurate picture of a DHH student.

> **CAUTION 5.4**
>
> Translation from English to ASL is not one-for-one. Examiners should understand that test item meaning could get lost when using an interpreter to administer standardized assessments to DHH young children.

AUTISM SPECTRUM DISORDER

Autism spectrum disorder (ASD) is a neurodevelopmental disorder that affects social interactions, communication, and behavior. Over the past two decades, the prevalence of ASD has changed dramatically, increasing from 1 in 150 children in 2000 to 1 in 44 children in 2018 (Maenner et al., 2021). According to the Office of Special Education Programs (United States Department of Education, 2020), ASD is the third largest educational disability category for preschool children ages 3–5, behind speech or language impairment and developmental delay. ASD was once considered a low incidence disorder; however, due to its increased prevalence, clinical and school psychologists more commonly receive referrals for differential diagnosis of ASD versus general developmental delays in very young children. Children with ASD display unique characteristics and needs that require targeted assessments. Many children with ASD require specialized medical, behavioral, and educational services, and early intervention is crucial. As a neurodevelopmental disorder, ASD manifests during early childhood. Its symptoms are often first recognized during the second year of life (12–24 months), and early diagnosis can confidently occur at 2 years old (Lord et al., 2006). Therefore, individuals who work with infants, toddlers, and preschoolers should be familiar with the symptoms of ASD and the assessments used to identify it. Accurate identification of

ASD occurs when a properly trained assessment professional utilizes clinical judgment informed by accurate assessment (Margiano et al., 2023). This section provides an overview of ASD assessment, and therefore, is not exhaustive.

Screeners

One approach for the early detection of ASD is screening. The American Academy of Pediatrics recommends that all children be screened for ASD at 18 and 24 months during regular well-child visits (Hyman et al., 2020). Screening tools include questionnaires and checklists that contain items related to the child's language, movement, language, and behavior (CDC, 2022). Some screeners are completed by parents, while others are interactive/observational measures administered by providers. There are multiple levels of screening to ensure all cases are captured and referral for a more comprehensive evaluation is made at the right time. It is important to note that screening tools do not automatically result in a diagnosis of ASD. That is, a child who fails a screening measure is not automatically diagnosed with ASD as some screeners have high false positive rates because they are designed to maximize sensitivity. Some of the most common screening tools are described below.

Level 1 Screeners

Level 1 screeners are universal measures administered to the general population. For example, these measures can be administered to all children within a primary care setting, preschool, or daycare.

- The Modified Checklist for Autism in Toddlers, Revised with Follow-Up (M-CHAT-R/F) is a two-stage parent-report screening tool (Robins et al., 2018). The M-CHAT-R/F is designed to screen for ASD in toddlers 16–30 months old. The first stage, which consists of 20 yes/no questions, takes approximately 5 minutes to administer and 2 minutes to score. If the screening is positive, the provider administers the second stage or refers the child for further evaluation.
- The Survey of Well-Being of Young Children (SWYC): Parent's Observations of Social Interactions (POSI) is a brief questionnaire that assesses the risk for ASD for children between the ages of 16 and 36 months. The questionnaire consists of seven items and takes approximately 5 minutes

for parents to complete. The POSI is one component of the SWYC, which assesses three domains of child functioning, including development, behavior, and family context (Smith et al., 2012).

Level 2 Screeners

Level 2 screeners are typically administered on children who have been identified as at-risk for ASD (e.g., having a sibling with ASD) or who scored positive on a Level 1 screener.

- The Screening Tool for Autism in Toddlers, and Young Children (STAT; Stone & Ousley, 2008) is a screener for children 24–36 months old who are suspected of having ASD. The STAT consists of 12 items completed by a trained provider, and it takes approximately 20 minutes to administer. Items are related to key social and communicative behavior often associated with ASD.
- The Rapid Interactive Screening Test for Autism in Toddlers (RITA-T; Choueiri & Wagner, 2015) is a play-based screener that can be administered to children 18–36 months old. The RITA-T assesses five different constructs, including joint attention, social awareness, awareness of human agency, self-recognition, and fundamental cognitive skill. It takes approximately 4–10 minutes to administer and score.
- The Social Communication Questionnaire (SCQ; Rutter et al., 2003a) and the Social Responsiveness Scale, Second Edition (SRS-2; Constantino, 2012) are two commonly used screening tools for ASD that are appropriate for young children. Both rating scales, ranging from 40 to 60 items, respectively, can be completed by a parent or teacher. The SCQ is based on the Autism Diagnostic Interview—Revised (ADI-R; Rutter et al., 2003b) algorithm and measures repetitive and stereotypes behaviors, communication, and reciprocal social interaction. Two forms are available: the Lifetime Form used to assess a child when the early developmental history is known, and the Current Form, which assesses behaviors that have occurred within the last 3 months. Items scored positively are indicative of autism, and a cut score of 15 or above should be referred for further assessment. The SRS-2 has a preschool form to use with children from 2.5 years to 4.5 years old, and a school-age form for children 4 and over. Results are presented as t-scores with greater elevations being more indicative of autism. A total severity score, as well as five subscales (Social Awareness,

Social Cognition, Social Communication, Social Motivation, and Autistic Mannerisms) are derived. Research has shown the SRS is a good tool to use to distinguish ASD from other childhood psychiatric illnesses and can be used as part of a comprehensive evaluation for a differential diagnosis (e.g., Duku et al., 2013).

• The Autism Spectrum Rating Scale (ASRS; Goldstein & Naglieri, 2009) is an ASD specific rating scale based on the diagnostic criteria of the DSM-5-TR. Young children from ages 2 through 5 years are rated by their parents and/or teacher on 70 behaviors associated with autism. The ASRS yields two summary scores (Total and DSM-5), two related to the diagnostic criteria of ASD (Social-Emotional Reciprocity), and eight treatment scales that can assist in intervention planning. Scores are presented as t-scores, with higher scores being more indicative of autism. Research suggests that the ASRS is helpful in differentiating ASD from intellectual disabilities (e.g., Li et al., 2018).

Diagnostic Tools

In cases where ASD is suspected, a comprehensive evaluation is warranted. Diagnostic tools, such as the Autism Diagnostic Observation Schedule, Second Edition (ADOS-2; Lord et al., 2012), are useful in eliciting behaviors related to ASD. The ADOS-2 consists of five modules, including a Toddler Module, which is administered to children 12–30 months of age. Modules 1 through 4 can be chosen based on the developmental language level of the child. A young child who is preverbal or uses single words and is over the age of 30 months can be administered Module 1 and those with phrase speech are administered Module 2. Examiners may also conduct a structured interview with the child's caregiver, using instruments such as the ADI-R; however, this tool may not be ideal for a clinical or educational setting due to the length of time it takes to administer.

Many children with ASD also experience developmental delays across a variety of domains, such as adaptive functioning, cognitive functioning, and motor skills. Although these domains are not diagnostic features, they can help identify concerns related to ASD. First, children with ASD experience pervasive and persistent deficits in adaptive functioning when compared to typically developing peers. A longitudinal study conducted by Franchini et al. (2018) found that young children with ASD demonstrated consistently lower adaptive functioning across all domains on the Vineland Adaptive Behavior Scales, Second Edition (Sparrow et al., 2005). In addition, young children with ASD tend to demonstrate lower scores on cognitive measures, such as the Bayley-4 Cognitive Scale (Dale et al., 2022). Research suggests there is a negative relationship between autism severity and cognitive functioning. For instance, higher scores on the ADOS-2 are associated with lower scores on the Bayley Scales of Infant and Toddler Development, Third Edition (Bayley-III; Bayley, 2006) Cognitive Scale (Ray-Subramanian et al., 2011). Although lower cognitive functioning is not always associated with ASD, roughly a third of children with ASD also have an intellectual disability (Maenner et al., 2021). Furthermore, motor skill deficits are also present in many children with ASD and may serve as one of the first signs of abnormal development. There is a negative relationship between motor skills and ASD severity scores, with lower fine and gross motor skills predicting more behaviors related to ASD symptomology (MacDonald et al., 2014).

Due to the developmental delays often seen in children with ASD, developmental measures may be particularly useful in screening infants and toddlers for ASD. One measure that has strong utility is the BDI-3, which is used from birth through 7 years, 11 months (Newborg, 2020). The BDI-3 assesses functioning in five domains, including communication, social/emotional, adaptive, motor, and cognitive development. Although research is still forthcoming on the BDI-3, there is a robust literature base demonstrating the relationship between the BDI-2 and ASD severity (Newborg, 2005). In studies involving the BDI-2, the Total Developmental Quotient (DQ) and Domain scores were statistically significant predictors of ASD screening outcomes, with the Personal-Social domain being the strongest predictor (Goldin et al., 2014; Peters & Matson, 2020). These findings suggest that the BDI-3 may be useful in screening for ASD in infants and toddlers. Furthermore, the Bayley-4 includes an ASD Checklist embedded across the Cognitive, Receptive Communication, and Expressive Communication subtests. Although independent research is not available on the validity of this tool, the inclusion of this screener in a broad developmental measure indicates the necessity of global screening tools for all children suspected of delays.

Social Developmental History/Clinical Interview

Examiners have many tools at their disposal to aid in the identification of ASD in young children. However, it is important to note that none of these tools can replace clinical judgment. A thorough social/developmental history is still the greatest tool available to diagnose ASD (Lord et al., 2006). Assessment specialists and special educators should immerse themselves in the field of autism to understand the full spectrum of abilities, signs, and symptoms. Examiners should conduct a thorough interview with parents, caregivers, and teachers to establish a consistent picture of the young child across settings. Although not exhaustive, Rapid Reference 5.6 lists several areas of development that should be covered in a structured developmental history.

≡ Rapid Reference 5.6 Sample Questions to Ask When Gathering a Social Developmental History

Early Development

Thinking back to when your child was an infant, would you describe them as fussy or easy?

Did your child extend their arms to indicate they wanted to be picked up?

Have you ever been concerned about your child's hearing?

Does your child enjoy games like peek-a-boo, patty cake, tickle monster, etc.?

Social Behaviors

How would you describe your child's eye contact? Do they look at you as you would expect?

Does it appear your child avoids making eye contact with others?

Does your child prefer to play alone over playing with peers?

Will your child allow you to join their play if you attempt to?

Does your child attempt to engage you in their play?

Will your child seek out peers to play with?

If another child attempts to play with your child, how do they react?

Does your child bring you things, like toys, or show you things?

Can your child imitate the actions of others?

Does your child act differently to strangers compared to those they know?

Communication

Did your child go through a babbling period?

How would you describe your child's vocabulary?

Prior to developing words, how did your child let you know their wants or needs?

Does your child point to reference a close or distant object?

Does your child look at you when requiring assistance?

When you call your child's name, do they respond? How?

Does your child ever repeat things they have heard others say or from the television?

Describe your child's back-and-forth conversation skills.

Interests and Repetitive Behaviors
What kind of toys does your child play with?

Does your child have a favorite object other than a toy?

Do they engage in imaginative or pretend play?

Have you ever noticed your child looking at objects out of the corner of their eye?

Is your child interested in parts of objects?

Does your child to the same thing over and over in their play?

Sensory Behaviors
Does your child appear fascinated with spinning objects?

Does your child try to hurt themselves through pinching, biting, head banging, etc.?

Describe your child's eating habits. Do they limit certain foods and prefer others?

How does your child react to pain?

Do any specific noises upset your child?

PRETERM BIRTH

Around the world, millions of infants are affected by preterm birth each year. Preterm birth occurs when a baby is born before the 37th week of pregnancy, and it is associated with a variety of health risks. In children under the age of 5, preterm birth complications are the leading cause of death, resulting in approximately one million deaths each year (Perin et al., 2021). It is important to note that not all preterm babies experience complications; however, the earlier the baby is born, the higher the risk of short-term and long-term complications. Some of these complications include low birth weight, anemia, breathing difficulties, heart problems, bleeding in the brain, jaundice, low blood pressure, and an increased risk of infection. In addition, preterm birth is associated with long-term complications such as cerebral palsy, impaired learning, vision and hearing problems, and developmental delays (Perin et al., 2021). Although preterm birth occurs spontaneously in many cases, it is also linked with a variety of prenatal risk factors, including multiple births (e.g., twins, triplets), chronic health conditions (e.g., diabetes and high blood pressure), and smoking cigarettes or using illicit substances during pregnancy.

It is worthwhile for examiners to be familiar with the preterm birth subcategories, as displayed in Rapid Reference 5.7. These subcategories are widely accepted conventions set forth by the World Health Organization (2022). However, researchers may encounter slightly different conventions in the literature.

≡ *Rapid Reference 5.7* Preterm Birth Subcategories

Moderate to Late Preterm	32–37 weeks
Very Preterm	28–32 weeks
Extremely Preterm	Less than 28 weeks

Children who are born preterm often receive early intervention services in infancy. Many of these services can be initiated by the neonatal intensive care unit staff before the infant is discharged to go home with the parents. In the preschool setting, although preterm birth is not considered an eligibility category under Part B of IDEA, children who are born prematurely may qualify for special education services due to a comorbid condition or general developmental delays. Examiners should be familiar with the educational and mental health outcomes associated with preterm birth. First, extremely preterm/very preterm (EP/VP) birth is linked with lower scores on cognitive tests (Winter et al., 2023). This relationship is evident during the infant and toddler periods and persists through preschool. One meta-analysis found that 3–5 year olds born before 32 weeks gestation scored 11.5 IQ points lower than their term-born peers (Arpi et al., 2019). Research also shows that this effect persists beyond preschool. For example, another meta-analysis found that children and adolescents (5 years–18 years old) scored almost one standard deviation (12.9 IQ points) lower than term-born controls (Twilhaar et al., 2018). Differences in cognitive abilities are most pronounced for those born extremely preterm, with one study finding that individuals born before 26 weeks gestation score 20 IQ points lower than their term-born peers (Johnson et al., 2009). Preterm birth is also associated with academic underachievement across a variety of measures. Compared to their term-born peers, preterm children score significantly lower on reading and math assessments, including those related to reading comprehension and applied math problems (McBryde et al., 2020). Preterm birth not only affects educational performance, but mental health outcomes as well. Children born preterm are at an increased risk of experiencing mental health problems, even from early childhood (Elgen et al., 2012). Accurate assessment of a young child's functional skills is imperative to assist in intervention planning and provide preterm infants and toddlers access to early intervention services.

CEREBRAL PALSY

Cerebral palsy is a group of lifelong disorders that impact a child's ability to move and maintain posture. It is also associated with disturbances of sensation (e.g., vision and hearing), perception, cognition, communication, and behavior, as well as an increased risk of epilepsy and secondary musculoskeletal problems (Rosenbaum et al., 2007). In the United States, cerebral palsy is the most common motor disability in childhood, with a prevalence of 2.9 per 1,000 children (Durkin et al., 2016). Cerebral palsy results from abnormal brain development or injury to the developing brain, such as genetic disorders, fetal stroke, and lack of oxygen during delivery. One of the leading risk factors for cerebral palsy is preterm birth, especially for babies born before 32 weeks gestation. There are several different types of cerebral palsy, including spastic cerebral palsy, dyskinetic cerebral palsy, ataxic cerebral palsy, and mixed cerebral palsy. The most common type is spastic cerebral palsy, which affects approximately 80% of children with cerebral palsy (Durkin et al., 2016). Spastic cerebral palsy is characterized by increased muscle tone, which results in jerky or exaggerated motor movements. The other types of cerebral palsy are associated with uncontrollable movement (dyskinesia) or poor balance and coordination (ataxia). Depending on the severity and type of cerebral palsy, mobility may be limited, although many people with cerebral palsy can walk independently or with a handheld mobility device (Durkin et al., 2016). The different types of cerebral palsy are listed in Rapid Reference 5.8.

Rapid Reference 5.8 Types of Cerebral Palsy

Type	Affected Brain Area	Symptoms
Spastic	Motor cortex	Jerky or exaggerated movements; increased muscle tone
Dyskinetic	Basal ganglia	Involuntary motor movements
Ataxic	Cerebellum	Shaky movements; poor balance and coordination
Mixed	Multiple areas	Combination of symptoms from other types

Source: Adapted from Durkin et al. (2016).

Cerebral palsy is typically diagnosed during the first 2 years of life (National Institute of Neurological Disorders and Stroke [NINDS], 2013). However, diagnosis may be delayed by several years if the child's symptoms are mild. To diagnose cerebral palsy, a medical provider evaluates the child's growth, development, and motor skills. Doctors may also use neuroimaging, such as a cranial ultrasound or magnetic resonance imaging (MRI), to detect abnormalities in the brain and rule out other possible causes. Due to overlapping symptomology, other disorders can be mistaken for cerebral palsy. For example, there are over 30 genetic and metabolic disorders that mimic the motor patterns associated with cerebral palsy (Hakami et al., 2019). One distinguishing characteristic that can aid in differential diagnosis is the nonprogressive nature of cerebral palsy. Although the exact symptoms may change, cerebral palsy does not become worse over time. If the child begins losing motor function, another disorder should be suspected. There is no cure for cerebral palsy, but the symptoms can be addressed through early intervention services, such as physical therapy, occupational therapy, and speech and language therapy.

For examiners, there are several factors to take into consideration when evaluating a young child with cerebral palsy. Like the other disabilities described in this chapter, no two individuals with cerebral palsy are exactly alike. Due to the different types and levels of severity, cerebral palsy represents a diverse group of individuals with varying strengths and needs. It is important to account for these strengths and needs before conducting an evaluation. For example, it is important to consider the child's fine and gross motor abilities. Many early childhood cognitive assessments, such as the WPPSI-IV, require the examinee to manipulate small objects (e.g., blocks and puzzle pieces), sometimes under time constraints. These tasks may be problematic for children with motor impairments, as they may have difficulty manipulating the objects. At that point, the task is no longer measuring what it is designed to measure, and it would be an unfair assessment of the child's cognitive abilities. For children with severe motor impairments, it is advisable to select tests with limited motor requirements. Scholars have identified several cognitive assessments that are suitable for use with the cerebral palsy population. For infants with cerebral palsy, there is empirical evidence supporting the use of the Mayes Motor-Free Compilation (Mayes, 1999) and

---

CAUTION 5.5

Selecting assessments that require the young child with cerebral palsy to utilize various manipulatives may result in an inaccurate assessment of skills.

an accommodated version of the Bayley Scales of Infant and Toddler Development (Morgan et al., 2019). In toddlers and preschoolers, recommended assessments include the Leiter International Performance Scale, the Peabody Picture Vocabulary Test, the Pictorial Test of Intelligence, and the Raven's Coloured Progressive Matrices (Yin Foo et al., 2013). Another viable solution is using select verbal measures, such as the Verbal Comprehension Index of the Wechsler Scales.

In addition to motor impairment, cerebral palsy can also affect cognition, vision, hearing, communication, and behavior. Cerebral palsy is associated with an increased risk of cognitive impairment. Although estimates vary, approximately 30–40% of individuals with cerebral palsy have an IQ of less than 70 (Stadskleiv, 2020). However, as described in the previous paragraph, careful test selection is needed to represent accurately the child's cognitive abilities. Furthermore, the examiner should consider if the standardization sample provides a fair basis for comparison.

SUMMARY OF LOW INCIDENCE DEVELOPMENTAL AND MEDICAL CONDITIONS

The assessment of special populations poses unique opportunities and challenges for examiners of young children. The remarkable heterogeneity represented by each population necessitates a highly individualized approach to assessment that considers the young child's strengths, abilities, and needs. Examiners are responsible for selecting tests and other assessment methods that can accurately capture the child's abilities.

Examiners are also encouraged to recognize their bounds of competence and seek consultation and continuing education when needed. The assessment of special populations often receives little attention in graduate training programs, and it is likely that examiners will encounter a population outside their expertise at one point or another. Interprofessional collaboration is essential when completing any comprehensive developmental evaluation of an infant, toddler, or preschooler; however, examiners may need to advocate for increased collaboration with special populations to ensure all their needs are assessed.

DON'T FORGET 5.4

Although this chapter provided a broad overview of low incidence developmental and medical disorders, it is not an exhaustive list. This chapter should be considered a starting point for examiners who work with these populations.

TEST YOURSELF

1. **Which of the following special populations could receive services under the Individuals with Disabilities Education Act (IDEA) Part C:**

   (a) Infants with a developmental delay

   (b) Toddlers with diagnosed physical condition that has a high probability of resulting in a developmental delay

   (c) Infants with a diagnosed mental condition that has a high probability of resulting in a developmental delay

   (d) All the above

2. **A child is referred to you due to difficulty with pragmatics in speech and slow sensorimotor development. When they come into your office, you notice they have a small jaw, broad forehead, short nose, and abnormal alignment of their eyes. Which syndrome best matches this child's features:**

   (a) Down Syndrome

   (b) Fragile X

   (c) Williams Syndrome

   (d) Angelman Syndrome

3. **Which document outlines all the medical services a child would need throughout their school day:**

   (a) Individualized Health Plan (IHP)

   (b) Individualized Education Plan (IEP)

   (c) Individualized Family Service Plan (IFSP)

   (d) None of the above

4. **The average age of onset for males with Fragile X is _______, whereas for females with Fragile X it is _______.**

   (a) 42 months (about 3 and a half years); 35 months (about 3 years)

   (b) 35 months (about 3 years); 42 months (about 3 and a half years)

   (c) 30 months (about 2 and a half years); 36 months (about 3 years)

   (d) 42 months (about 3 and a half years); 28 months (about 2 and a half years)

5. **Which of the following are ways to identify Down Syndrome during pregnancy:**

   (a) Prenatal screenings

   (b) Blood testing

(c) Ultrasounds

(d) All the above

6. **In Turner's Syndrome, which chromosome is damaged:**

(a) Y chromosome

(b) Chromosome 21

(c) X chromosome

(d) All the above

7. **A female presents with short stature, premature ovarian failure, and a "webbed" neck. Which syndrome best matches this child's features:**

(a) Turner's Syndrome

(b) Angelman Syndrome

(c) Down Syndrome

(d) Fragile X

8. **An individual presents with a protruding tongue, deep-set eyes, prominent chin, and frequent drooling. Parents report that they did not start walking till they were 4 years old and can only say a few words. Which syndrome best matches this child's features:**

(a) Down Syndrome

(b) Fragile X

(c) Angelman Syndrome

(d) Turner's Syndrome

9. **A psychologist is evaluating a 4 year old for intellectual developmental disorder (IDD). The psychologist is not confident in the standardized testing results due to the child's limited ability to participate in testing. According to the DSM-5-TR, what other disorder could the psychologist consider:**

(a) Developmental Coordination Disorder

(b) Global Developmental Disorder

(c) Speech Pragmatic Disorder

(d) None of the above

10. **What is the recommended age to start interventions for individuals diagnosed with hearing loss:**

(a) 6 months

(b) 12 months

(c) 18 months

(d) 32 months

Answers: 1. d; 2. c; 3. a; 4. b; 5. d; 6. c; 7. a; 8. c; 9. b; 10. a

REFERENCES

Abbeduto, L., & Murphy, M. M. (2004). Language, social cognition, maladaptive behavior, and communication in Down syndrome and fragile X syndrome. In M. L. Rice & S. F. Warren (Eds.), *Developmental language disorders: From phenotypes to etiologies* (pp. 77–97). Erlbaum.

American Psychiatric Association. (2022). *Diagnostic and statistical manual of mental disorders* (5th ed., text rev.). Author. https://doi.org/10.1176/appi.books.9780890425787

Andersen, W. H., Rasmussen, R. K., & Strømme, P. (2001). Levels of cognitive and linguistic development in Angelman syndrome: A study of 20 children. *Logopedics, Phoniatrics, Vocology, 26*(1), 2–9. https://doi.org/10.1080/14015430117324

Anderson, V. A., Morse, S. A., Catroppa, C., Haritou, F., & Rosenfeld, J. V. (2004). Thirty month outcome from early childhood head injury: A prospective analysis of neurobehavioural recovery. *Brain, 127*(12), 2608–2620. https://doi.org/10.1093/brain/awh320

Araki, T., Yokota, H., & Morita, A. (2017). Pediatric traumatic brain injury: Characteristic features, diagnosis, and management. *Neurologia Medico-Chirurgica, 57*(2), 82–93. https://doi.org/10.2176/nmc.ra.2016-0191

Arora, P., Levine, J., & Goldstein, T. (2019). School psychologists' interprofessional collaboration with medical providers: An initial examination of training, preparedness, and current practices. *Psychology in the Schools, 56*(4), 554–568. https://doi.org/10.1002/pits.22208

Arpi, E., D'Amico, R., Lucaccioni, L., Bedetti, L., Berardi, A., & Ferrari, F. (2019). Worse global intellectual and worse neuropsychological functioning in preterm-born children at preschool age: A meta-analysis. *Acta Paediatrica, 108*(9), 1567–1579. https://doi.org/10.1111/apa.14836

Backes, M., Genc, B., Schreck, J., Doerfler, W., Lehmkuhl, G., & Von Gontard, A. (2000). Cognitive and behavioral profile of fragile X boys: Correlations to molecular data. *American Journal of Medical Genetics, 95*(2), 150–156. https://doi.org/ 10.1002/1096-8628(20001113)95:23.0.CO;2-1

Bailey, D. B., Jr., Raspa, M., Olmsted, M., & Holiday, D. B. (2008). Co-occurring conditions associated with FMR1 gene variations: Findings from a national parent survey. *American Journal of Medical Genetics. Part A, 146A*(16), 2060–2069. https://doi.org/10.1002/ajmg.a.32439

Bailey, D. B., Raspa, M., Bishop, E., & Holiday, D. (2009). No change in the age of diagnosis for fragile X syndrome: Findings from a national parent survey. *Pediatrics, 124*(2), 527–533. https://doi.org/10.1542/peds.2008-2992

Bartholomay, K. L., Lee, C. H., Bruno, J. L., Lightbody, A. A., & Reiss, A. L. (2019). Closing the gender gap in fragile X syndrome: Review of females with fragile X syndrome and preliminary research findings. *Brain Sciences, 9*(1), 11. https://doi.org/10.3390/brainsci9010011

Bayley, N. (2006). *Bayley scales of infant and toddler development, third edition: Administration manual*. Harcourt.

Bayley, N., & Aylward, G. P. (2019). *Bayley-4: Scales of infant and toddler development, Technical manual* (4th ed.). Pearson.

Berry-Kravis, E. (2002). Epilepsy in fragile X syndrome. *Developmental Medicine and Child Neurology, 44*(11), 724–728. https://doi.org/10.1017/S0012162201002833

Berry-Kravis, E., Knox, A., & Hervey, C. (2011). Targeted treatments for fragile X syndrome. *Journal of Neurodevelopmental Disorders, 3*(3), 193–210. https://doi.org/10.1007/ s11689-011-9074-7

Boat, T. F., Wu, J. T., & National Academies of Sciences, Engineering, and Medicine. (2015). Clinical characteristics of intellectual disabilities. In T. F. Boat & J. T. Wu (Eds.), *Mental disorders and disabilities among low-income children* (pp. 169–178). National Academies Press. Retrieved December 6, 2022 from https://www.ncbi.nlm.nih.gov/books/NBK332877/.

Bracken, B. A. (1987). Limitations of preschool instruments and standards for minimal levels of technical adequacy. *Journal of Psychoeducational Assessment, 5*(4), 313–326.

Bradley-Johnson, S. (2001). Cognitive assessment for the youngest children: A critical review of tests. *Journal of Psychoeducational Assessment, 19*(1), 19–44. https://doi. org/10.1177/073428290101900102

Bruce, S. M., Bashinski, S. M., Covelli, A. J., Bernstein, V., Zatta, M. C., & Briggs, S. (2018). Positive behavior supports for individuals who are deafblind with CHARGE syndrome. *Journal of Visual Impairment & Blindness, 112*(5), 497–560. https://doi.org/10.1177/0145482X11200507

Bull, M. J., Saal, H. M., Braddock, S. R., Enns, G. M., Gruen, J. R., Perrin, J. M., Saul, R. A., & Tarini, B. (2011). Health supervision for children with Down syndrome. *Pediatrics, 128*(2), 393–406. https://doi.org/10.1542/peds.2011-1605

Centers for Disease Control and Prevention. (2022). Screening and diagnosis of autism spectrum disorder. Retrieved February 7, 2023 from https://www.cdc.gov/ncbddd/autism/screening.html.

Centers for Disease Control and Prevention. (2021). *Facts about down syndrome.* Centers for Disease Control and Prevention. Retrieved February 7, 2023 from https://www.cdc.gov/ncbddd/birthdefects/downsyndrome.html.

Choueiri, R., & Wagner, S. (2015). A new interactive screening test for autism spectrum disorders in toddlers. *Journal of Pediatrics, 167*(2), 460–466.

Clayton-Smith, J., & Laan, L. A. E. M. (2003). Angelman syndrome: A review of the clinical and genetic aspects. *Journal of Medical Genetics, 40*(2), 87–95. https://doi.org/10.1136/jmg.40.2.87

Clayton-Smith, J., & Pembrey, M. E. (1992). Angelman syndrome. *Journal of Medical Genetics, 29*(6), 412.

Cleveland Clinic. (2021a). *Genetic disorders: What are they, types, symptoms & causes.* Cleveland Clinic. Retrieved December 6, 2022 from https://my.clevelandclinic.org/health/diseases/21751-genetic-disorders.

Cleveland Clinic. (2021b). Turner syndrome: Causes, symptoms, diagnosis & treatment. Retrieved December 6, 2022 from https://my.clevelandclinic.org/health/diseases/15200-turner-syndrome.

Constantino, J. N. (2012). *Social responsiveness scale* (2nd ed.). Western Psychological Services.

Coplan, J. (1993). *Early language milestone scale-2.* Pro-Ed.

Corona, L. L., Wagner, L., Wade, J., Weitlauf, A. S., Hine, J., Nicholson, A., Stone, C., Vehorn, A., & Warren, Z. (2021). Toward novel tools for autism identification: Fusing computational and clinical expertise. *Journal of Autism and Developmental Disorders, 51*, 4003–4012. https://doi.org/10.1007/s10803-020-04857-x

Costa, E. B. A., Day, L. A., & Raiford, S. E. (2015). Testing children who are deaf or hard of hearing (WPPSI–IV Technical Report #1). Bloomington, MN: NCS, Pearson, Inc. Retrieved January 22, 2023 from http://images.pearsonclinical.com/images/Products/WPPSIIV/WPPSI%E2%80%93IVTechReport_1_FNL.pdf.

Dale, B. A., Caemmerer, J. M., Winter, E. L., & Kaufman, A. S. (2022). Bayley-4 performance of very young children with autism, developmental delay, and language impairment. *Psychology in the Schools, 59.* https://doi.org/10.1002/pits.22682

Dale, B. A., & Neild, R. (2020). Assessment of co-occurring disabilities in young children who are deaf and hard of hearing. *Perspectives on Early Childhood Psychology and Education, 5*(2), 219–241. https://doi.org/10.1002/pits.22328

De Vries, B. B., Wiegers, A. M., Smits, A. P., Mohkamsing, S., Duivenvoorden, H. J., Fryns, J. P., Curfs, L. M., Halley, D. J., Oostra, B. A., van den Ouweland, A. M., & Niermeijer, M. F. (1996). Mental status of females with an FMR1 gene full mutation. *American Journal of Human Genetics, 58*(5), 1025. Retrieved December 6, 2022 from https://www.ncbi.nlm.nih.gov/pmc/articles/PMC1914633/.

Diedrichsen, J., Shadmehr, R., & Ivry, R. B. (2010). The coordination of movement: Optimal feedback control and beyond. *Trends in Cognitive Sciences, 14*(1), 31–39. https://doi.org/10.1016/j.tics.2009.11.004

Diez-Itza, E., Viejo, A., & Fernández-Urquiza, M. (2022). Pragmatic profiles of adults with fragile X syndrome and Williams syndrome. *Brain Sciences, 12*(3), 385. https://doi.org/10.3390/brainsci12030385

van Dijk, R., Nelson, C., Postma, A., & van Dijk, J. (2010). Deaf children with severe multiple disabilities: Etiologies, intervention, and assessment. *The Oxford Handbook of Deaf Studies, Language, and Education, 2*, 172–191.

Duku, E., Vaillancourt, T., Szatmari, P., Georgiades, S., Zwaigenbaum, L., Smith, I. M., Bryson, S., Fombonne, E., Miranda, P., Roberts, W., Volden, J., Waddell, C., Thompson, A., Bennett, T., & Pathways in ASD Study Team. (2013). Investigating the measurement properties of the social responsiveness scale in preschool children with autism spectrum disorders. *Journal of Autism and Developmental Disorders, 43*, 860–868. https://doi.org/10.1007/s10803-012-1627-4

Durkin, M. S., Benedict, R. E., Christensen, D., Dubois, L. A., Fitzgerald, R. T., Kirby, R. S., Maenner, M. J., Van Naarden Braun, K., Wingate, M. S., & Yeargin-Allsopp, M. (2016). Prevalence of cerebral palsy among 8-year-old children in 2010 and preliminary evidence of trends in its relationship to low birthweight. *Paediatric and Perinatal Epidemiology, 30*(5), 496–510. https://doi.org/10.1111/ppe.12299

Early Hearing Detection & Intervention. (2022). EHDI legislation: Overview. Retrieved January 22, 2023 from https://www.infanthearing.org/legislation/.

Elgen, S. K., Leversen, K. T., Grundt, J. H., Hurum, J., Sundby, A. B., Elgen, I. B., & Markestad, T. (2012). Mental health at 5 years among children born extremely preterm: A national population-based study. *European Child & Adolescent Psychiatry, 21*(10), 583–589. https://doi.org/10.1007/s00787-012-0298-1

Ewing-Cobbs, L., Fletcher, J. M., Levin, H. S., Francis, D. J., Davidson, K., & Miner, M. E. (1997). Longitudinal neuropsychological outcome in infants and preschoolers with traumatic brain injury. *Journal of the International Neuropsychological Society, 3*(6), 581–591. https://doi.org/10.1017/S1355617779700581X

Franchini, M., Zöller, D., Gentaz, E., Glaser, B., Wood de Wilde, H., Kojovic, N., Eliez, S., & Schaer, M. (2018). Early adaptive functioning trajectories in preschoolers with autism spectrum disorders. *Journal of Pediatric Psychology, 43*(7), 800–813. https://doi.org/10.1093/jpepsy/jsy024

Friefeld, S. J., & Macgregor, D. (1994). Sensorimotor coordination in boys with fragile X syndrome. *Occupational Therapy International, 1*, 174–182. https://doi.org/10.1002/oti.6150010305

Goldin, R. L., Matson, J. L., Beighley, J. S., & Jang, J. (2014). Autism spectrum disorder severity as a predictor of Battelle Developmental Inventory–Second Edition (BDI-2) scores in toddlers. *Developmental Neurorehabilitation, 17*(1), 39–43. https://doi.org/10.3109/17518423.2013.839585

Goldstein, S., & Naglieri, J. A. (2009). *ASRS: Autism Spectrum Rating Scales*. Multi-Health Systems.

Gothelf, D., Farber, N., Raveh, E., Apter, A., & Attias, J. (2006). Hyperacusis in Williams syndrome: Characteristics and associated neuroaudiologic abnormalities. *Neurology, 66*(3), 390–395. https://doi.org/10.1212/01.wnl.0000196643.35395.5f

Gravholt, C. H., Andersen, N. H., Conway, G. S., Dekkers, O. M., Geffner, M. E., Klein, K. O., Lin, A. E., Mauras, N., Quigley, C. A., Rubin, K., Sandberg, D. E., Sas, T. C. J., Silberbach, M., Söderström-Anttila, V., Stochholm, K., van Alfen-van derVelden, J. A., Woelfle, J., Backeljauw, P. F., & International Turner Syndrome Consensus Group. (2017). Clinical practice guidelines for the care of girls and women with turner syndrome: Proceedings from the 2016 cincinnati international turner syndrome meeting. *European Journal of Endocrinology, 177*(3), G1–G70. https://doi.org/10.1530/EJE-17-0430

Grieco, J., Pulsifer, M., Seligsohn, K., Skotko, B., & Schwartz, A. (2015). Down syndrome: Cognitive and behavioral functioning across the lifespan. *American Journal of Medical Genetics. Part C, Seminars in Medical Genetics, 169*(2), 135–149. https://doi.org/10.1002/ajmg.c.31439

Haarbauer-Krupa, J., Haileyesus, T., Gilchrist, J., Mack, K. A., Law, C. S., & Joseph, A. (2019). Fall-related traumatic brain injury in children ages 0–4 years. *Journal of Safety Research, 70*, 127–133. https://doi.org/10.1016/j.jsr.2019.06.003

Hagerman, R. (1999). *Neurodevelopmental disorders*. Oxford University Press.

Hagerman, R. (2002). The physical and behavioral phenotype. In R. J. Hagerman & P. J. Hagerman (Eds.), *Fragile X syndrome: Diagnosis, treatment, and research* (3rd ed., pp. 1–109). Johns Hopkins University Press.

Hagerman, R. J., Jackson, C., Amiri, K., Silverman, A. C., O'Connor, R., & Sobesky, W. (1992). Girls with fragile X syndrome: Physical and neurocognitive status and outcome. *Pediatrics, 89*(3), 395–400. https://doi.org/10.1542/peds.89.3.395

Hakami, W. S., Hundallah, K. J., & Tabarki, B. M. (2019). Metabolic and genetic disorders mimicking cerebral palsy. *Neurosciences (Riyadh, Saudi Arabia), 24*(3), 155–163. https://doi.org/10.17712/nsj.2019.3.20190045

Hall, W. C., Levin, L. L., & Anderson, M. L. (2017). Language deprivation syndrome: A possible neurodevelopmental disorder with sociocultural origins. *Social Psychiatry and Psychiatric Epidemiology, 52,* 761–776. https://doi.org/10.1007/s00127-017-1351-7

Hall, S. S., Lightbody, A. A., & Reiss, A. L. (2008). Compulsive, self-injurious, and autistic behavior in children and adolescents with fragile X syndrome. *American Journal on Mental Retardation, 113*(1), 44–53.

Hall, S. S., Maynes, N. P., & Reiss, A. L. (2009). Using percentile schedules to increase eye contact in children with fragile X syndrome. *Journal of Applied Behavior Analysis, 42*(1), 171–176. https://doi.org/10.1901/jaba.2009.42-171

Hatton, D. D., Sideris, J., Skinner, M., Mankowski, J., Bailey, D. B., Jr., Roberts, J., & Mirrett, P. (2006). Autistic behavior in children with fragile X syndrome: Prevalence, stability, and the impact of FMRP. *American Journal of Medical Genetics Part A, 140*(17), 1804–1813. https://doi.org/10.1002/ajmg.a.31286

Hyman, S. L., Levy, S. E., & Myers, S. M. (2020). Executive summary: Identification, evaluation, and management of children with autism spectrum disorder. *Pediatrics, 145*(1). https://doi.org/10.1542/peds.2019-3448

Individuals With Disabilities Education Act, 20 U.S.C. § 1400 (2004).

Jarrold, C., Nadel, L., & Vicari, S. (2008). Memory and neuropsychology in Down syndrome. *Down Syndrome: Research & Practice, 12*(3), 196–201. https://doi.org/10.3104/reviews.2068

Johnson, S., Hennessy, E., Smith, R., Trikic, R., Wolke, D., & Marlow, N. (2009). Academic attainment and special educational needs in extremely preterm children at 11 years of age: The EPICure study. *Archives of Disease in Childhood-Fetal and Neonatal Edition, 94*(4), F283–F289. https://doi.org/10.1136/adc.2008.152793

Joyce, T., Gossman, W., & Huecker, M. R. (2022). *Pediatric abusive head trauma.* StatPearls. Stat Pearls Publishing.

Karam, S. M., Barros, A. J. D., Matijasevich, A., dos Santos, I. S., Anselmi, L., Barros, F., Leistner-Segal, S., Félix, T. M., Riegel, M., Maluf, S. W., Giugliani, R., & Black, M. M. (2016). Intellectual disability in a birth cohort: Prevalence, etiology, and determinants at the age of 4 years. *Public Health Genomics, 19*(5), 290–297. https://doi.org/10.1159/000448912

Kerins, M. (2018). Promoting interprofessional practice in schools. American Speech-Hearing-Language Association. *Leadership, 23*(12), 32–33. https://doi.org/10.1044/leader.SCM.23122018.32

Keysor, C. S., & Mazzocco, M. M. (2002). A developmental approach to understanding fragile X syndrome in females. *Microscopy Research and Technique, 57*(3), 179–186. https://doi.org/10.1002/jemt.10070

Kriel, R. L., Krach, L. E., & Panser, L. A. (1989). Closed head injury: Comparison of children younger and older than 6 years of age. *Pediatric Neurology, 5*(5), 296–300. https://doi.org/10.1016/0887-8994(89)90021-0

Kronk, R., Bishop, E. E., Raspa, M., Bickel, J. O., Mandel, D. A., & Bailey, D. B., Jr. (2010). Prevalence, nature, and correlates of sleep problems among children with fragile X syndrome based on a large scale parent survey. *Sleep, 33*(5), 679–687. https://doi.org/10.1093/sleep/33.5.679

Kronk, R., Dahl, R., & Noll, R. (2009). Caregiver reports of sleep problems on a convenience sample of children with fragile X syndrome. *American Journal on Intellectual and Developmental Disabilities, 114*(6), 383–392. https://doi.org/10.1352/1944-7588-114.6.383

Kruzliakova, N. A., Dale, B., Remache, L. J., McIntosh, C. E., & Kandiah, J. (2021). Interprofessional collaboration in school-based settings, part 3: Implementation of IC through case scenarios. *NASN School Nurse, 36*(5), 271–275. https://doi.org/10.1177/19426X211008639

Lachiewicz, A. M., Dawson, D. V., Spiridigliozzi, G. A., & McConkie-Rosell, A. (2006). Arithmetic difficulties in females with the fragile X premutation. *American Journal of Medical Genetics Part A, 140*(7), 665–672. https://doi.org/10.1002/ajmg.a.31082

Lange-Cosack, H., Wider, B., Schlesner, H. J., Grumme, T., & Kubicki, S. (1979). Prognosis of brain injuries in young children (one until five years of age). *Neuropaediatrie, 10*(2), 105–127. https://doi.org/10.1055/s-0028-1085318

Leppo, R. H. T., Cawthon, S. W., & Bond, M. P. (2014). Including deaf and hard-of-hearing students with co-occurring disabilities in the accommodations discussion. *Journal of Deaf Studies and Deaf Education, 19*(2), 189–202. https://doi.org/10.1093/deafed/ent029

Leyfer, O. T., Woodruff-Borden, J., Klein-Tasman, B. P., Fricke, J. S., & Mervis, C. B. (2006). Prevalence of psychiatric disorders in 4 to 16-year-olds with Williams syndrome. *American Journal of Medical Genetics Part B: Neuropsychiatric Genetics, 141*(6), 615–622. https://doi.org/10.1002/ajmg.b.30344

Li, C., Zhou, H., Wang, T., Long, S., Du, X., Xu, X., Yan, W., & Wang, Y. Performance of the Autim Spectrum Rating Scale and the Social Reponsiveness Scale in identifying autism spectrum disorder among cases of intellectual disability. *Neuropsychological Bulletin, 34*, 972–980. https://doi.org/10.1007/s12264-018-0237-3

Lippe, B., Geffner, M. E., Dietrich, R. B., Boechat, M. I., & Kangarloo, H. (1988). Renal malformations in patients with Turner syndrome: Imaging in 141 patients. *Pediatrics, 82*(6), 852–856. https://doi.org/10.1542/peds.82.6.852

Lord, C., Luyster, R. J., Gotham, K., & Guthrie, W. (2012). *Autism diagnostic observation schedule, second edition (ADOS-2) manual (Part II): Toddler module.* Western Psychological Services.

Lord, C., Risi, S., DiLavore, P. S., Shulman, C., Thurm, A., & Pickles, A. (2006). Autism from 2 to 9 years of age. *Archives of General Psychiatry, 63*(6), 694–701. https://doi.org/10.1001/archpsyc.63.6.694

Lyness, C. R., Woll, B., Campbell, R., & Cardin, V. (2013). How does visual language affect crossmodal plasticity and cochlear implant success? *Neuroscience & Biobehavioral Reviews, 37*, 2621–2630. https://doi.org/10.1016/j.neubiorev.2013.08.011

MacDonald, M., Lord, C., & Ulrich, D. A. (2014). Motor skills and calibrated autism severity in young children with autism spectrum disorder. *Adapted Physical Activity Quarterly, 31*(2), 95–105. https://doi.org/10.1123/apaq.2013-0068

Maenner, M. J., Shaw, K. A., Bakian, A. V., Bilder, D. A., Durkin, M. S., Esler, A., … Cogswell, M. E. (2021). Prevalence and characteristics of autism spectrum disorder among children aged 8 years–autism and developmental disabilities monitoring network, 11 sites, United States, 2018. *MMWR Surveillance Summaries, 70*(11), 1–16. https://doi.org/10.15585/mmwr.ss7011a1

Mai, C. T., Isenburg, J. L., Canfield, M. A., Meyer, R. E., Correa, A., Alverson, C. J., Lupo, P. J., Riehle-Colarusso, T., Cho, S. J., Aggarwal, D., Kirby, R. S., & Network, N. B. D. P. (2019). National population-based estimates for major birth defects, 2010–2014. *Birth Defects Research, 111*(18), 1420–1435. https://doi.org/10.1002/bdr2.1589

Malak, R., Kotwicka, M., Krawczyk-Wasielewska, A., Mojs, E., & Szamborski, W. (2013). Motor skills, cognitive development and balance functions of children with Down syndrome. *Annals of Agricultural and Environmental Medicine, 20*(4), 803–806.

Margiano, S. G., Sassu, K. A., Dale, B. A., Caemmerer, J. M., & Bray, M. A. (2023). School psychologists and autism identification: Present challenges and potential solutions. *Psychology in the Schools, 60*, 441–451. https://doi.org/10.1002/pits.22799

Margolis, S. S., Sell, G. L., Zbinden, M. A., & Bird, L. M. (2015). Angelman syndrome. *Neurotherapeutics, 12*(3), 641–650. https://doi.org/10.1007/s13311-015-0361-y

Markelz, A. M., & Batement, D. F. (2021). *The essentials of special education law*. Rowman & Littlefield Publishers.

Martin, G. E., Roberts, J. E., Helm-Estabrooks, N., Sideris, J., Vanderbilt, J., & Moskowitz, L. (2012). Perseveration in the connected speech of boys with fragile X syndrome with and without autism spectrum disorder. *American Journal on Intellectual and Developmental Disabilities, 117*(5), 384–399. https://doi.org/10.1352/1944-7558-117.5.384

Mayes, S. M. (1999). Mayes motor-free compilation (MMFC) for assessing mental ability in children with physical impairments. *International Journal of Disability, Development and Education, 46*, 475–485. https://doi.org/10.1080/103491299100452

Mazzocco, M. M. (2006). The cognitive phenotype of Turner syndrome: Specific learning disabilities. *International Congress Series, 1298*, 83–92. https://doi.org/10.1016/j.ics.2006.06.016

McBryde, M., Fitzallen, G. C., Liley, H. G., Taylor, H. G., & Bora, S. (2020). Academic outcomes of school-aged children born preterm: A systematic review and meta-analysis. *JAMA Network Open, 3*(4). https://doi.org/10.1001/jamanetworkopen.2020.2027

McIntosh, C. E., Dale, B., Kruzliakova, N., & Kandiah, J. (2021). Interprofessional collaboration in school-based settings part 1: Definition and the role of the school nurse. *NASN School Nurse, 36*(3), 170–175. https://doi.org/10.1177/1942602X20985420

McLaren, J., & Bryson, S. E. (1987). Review of recent epidemiological studies of mental retardation: Prevalence, associated disorders, and etiology. *American Journal on Mental Retardation, 92*(3), 243–254.

Mertz, L. G. B., Christensen, R., Vogel, I., Hertz, J. M., Nielsen, K. B., Grønskov, K., & Østergaard, J. R. (2013). Angelman syndrome in Denmark. Birth incidence, genetic findings, and age at diagnosis. *American Journal of Medical Genetics Part A, 161*(9), 2197–2203. https://doi.org/10.1002/ajmg.a.36058

Mervis, C. B., & Morris, C. A. (2007). Williams syndrome. In M. M. Mazzocco & J. L. Ross (Eds.), *Neurogenetic developmental disorders: Variation of manifestation in childhood* (pp. 199–262). Massachusetts Institute of Technology.

Mervis, C. B., Robinson, B. F., Rowe, M. L., Becerra, A. M., & Klein Tasman, B. P. (2003). Language abilities of individuals with Williams syndrome. In L. Abbeduto (Ed.), *International review of research in mental retardation, 27* (pp. 35–81). Academic Press.

Mervis, C. B., & Velleman, S. L. (2011). Children with Williams syndrome: Language, cognitive, and behavioral characteristics and their implications for intervention. *Perspectives on Language Learning and Education, 18*(3), 98–107. https://doi.org/10.1044/lle18.3.98

Miclea, D., Peca, L., Cuzmici, Z., & Pop, I. V. (2015). Genetic testing in patients with global developmental delay/intellectual disabilities. A review. *Clujul Medical, 88*(3), 288–292. https://doi.org/10.15386/cjmed-461

Miles, B. (2008). Overview on deaf-blindness. *The National Information Clearinghouse on Children who are Deaf-Blind*. Retrieved January 22, 2023 from https://www.nationaldb.org/info-center/overview-factsheet/.

Mirrett, P. L., Bailey, D. B., Jr., Roberts, J. E., & Hatton, D. D. (2004). Developmental screening and detection of developmental delays in infants and toddlers with fragile X syndrome. *Journal of Developmental & Behavioral Pediatrics, 25*(1), 21–27. https://doi.org/10.1097/00004703-200402000-00004

Morgan, C., Honan, I., Allsop, A., Novak, I., & Badawi, N. (2019). Psychometric properties of assessments of cognition in infants with cerebral palsy or motor impairment: A systematic review. *Journal of Pediatric Psychology, 44*(2), 238–252. https://doi.org/10.1093/jpepsy/jsy068

Morris, C. A. (2010). Introduction: Williams syndrome. *American Journal of Medical Genetics. Part C, Seminars in Medical Genetics, 154*(2), 203–208. https://doi.org/10.1002/ajmg.c.30266

Moss, J., & Howlin, P. (2009). Autism spectrum disorders in genetic syndromes: Implications for diagnosis, intervention and understanding the wider autism spectrum disorder population. *Journal of Intellectual Disability Research, 53*(10), 852–873. https://doi.org/10.1111/j.1365-2788.2009.01197.x

National Association of School Nurses. (2020). *Use of individualized healthcare plans to support school health services (Position Statement)*. Author.

National Association of School Psychologists. (2020). Position statement: Serving students who are deaf or hard of hearing. Retrieved February 7, 2023 from https://www.nasponline.org/research-and-policy/policy-priorities/position-statements/serving-deaf-and-hard-of-hearing-students-and-their-families-implications-for-education-and-service-delivery.

National Center on Deaf-Blindness. (2020). 2019 National deaf-blind child count. Retrieved February 7, 2023 from https://www.nationaldb.org/products/national-child-count/report-2019.

National Institute of Neurological Disorders and Stroke. (2013). Cerebral palsy: Hope through research. Retrieved December 6, 2022 from https://www.ninds.nih.gov/Disorders/Patient-Caregiver-Education/Hope-Through-Research/Cerebral-Palsy-Hope-Through-Research.

Newborg, J. (2005). *Battelle developmental inventory* (2nd ed.). In *Examiner's Manual)*. Riverside Publishing. 240

Newborg, J. (2020). *Battelle developmental inventory* (3rd ed.). In *Examiner's Manual)*. Riverside Publishing.

Nicholas, J. (2020). Cognitive assessment of children who are deafblind: Perspectives and suggestions for assessments. *Frontiers in Psychology, 11*, 571358. https://doi.org/10.3389/fpsyg.2020.571358

Onnivello, S., Pulina, F., Locatelli, C., Marcolin, C., Ramacieri, G., Antonaros, F., Vione, B., Caracausi, M., & Lanfranchi, S. (2022). Cognitive profiles in children and adolescents with Down syndrome. *Scientific Reports, 12*(1), 1–14. https://doi.org/10.1038/s41598-022-05825-4

Patel, D. R., Cabral, M. D., Ho, A., & Merrick, J. (2020). A clinical primer on intellectual disability. *Translational Pediatrics, 9*(Suppl 1), S23–S35. https://doi.org/10.21037/tp.2020.02.02

Patterson, D. (2007). Genetic mechanisms involved in the phenotype of Down syndrome. *Mental Retardation and Developmental Disabilities Research Reviews, 13*(3), 199–206. https://doi.org/10.1002/mrdd.20162

Pelc, K., Cheron, G., Boyd, S. G., & Dan, B. (2008). Are there distinctive sleep problems in Angelman syndrome? *Sleep Medicine, 9*(4), 434–441. https://doi.org/10.1016/j.sleep.2007.07.001

Perin, J., Mulick, A., Yeung, D., Villavicencio, F., Lopez, G., Strong, K. L., Prieto-Merino, D., Cousens, S., Black, R. E., & Liu, L. (2021). Global, regional, and national causes of under-5 mortality in 2000–19: an updated systematic analysis with implications for the Sustainable Development Goals. *The Lancet Child & Adolescent Health, 6*(2), 106–115. https://doi.org/10.1016/S2352-4642(21)00311-4

Peters, W. J., & Matson, J. L. (2020). The relationship between developmental functioning and screening outcome for autism spectrum disorder. *Journal of Developmental and Physical Disabilities, 32*(2), 293–305. https://doi.org/10.1007/s10882-019-09689-x

Pezzini, G., Vicari, S., Volterra, V., Milani, L., & Ossella, M. T. (1999). Children with Williams syndrome: Is there a single neuropsychological profile? *Developmental Neuropsychology, 15*(1), 141–155. https://doi.org/10.1080/87565649909540742

Ray-Subramanian, C. E., Huai, N., & Ellis Weismer, S. (2011). Brief report: Adaptive behavior and cognitive skills for toddlers on the autism spectrum. *Journal of Autism and Developmental Disorders, 41*(5), 679–684. https://doi.org/10.1007/s10803-010-1083-y

Rhodes, S., Riby, D., Matthews, K., & Coghill, D. (2011). Attention-deficit/hyperactivity disorder and Williams syndrome: Shared behavioral and neuropsychological profiles. *Journal of Clinical and Experimental Neuropsychology, 33*(1), 147–156. https://doi.org/10.1080/13803395.2010.495057

Robins, D. L., Fein, D., & Barton, M. (2018). *Modified checklist for autism in toddlers, revised, with follow-up (M-CHAT-R/F) TM*. LineageN.

Robinson, A., Bender, B. G., & Linden, M. G. (1990). Summary of clinical findings in children and young adults with sex chromosome anomalies. *Birth Defects Original Article Series, 26*(4), 225–228.

Rosenbaum, P., Paneth, N., Leviton, A., Goldstein, M., Bax, M., Damiano, D., … Jacobsson, B. (2007). A report: The definition and classification of cerebral palsy April 2006. *Developmental Medicine and Child Neurology. Supplement, 109*(suppl 109), 8–14.

Rourke, B. P. (1995). *Syndrome of nonverbal learning disabilities: Neurodevelopmental manifestations*. The Guilford Press.

Rowland, C. (2009). Assessing communication and learning in young children who are deafblind or who have multiple disabilities. Retrieved January 22, 2023 from https://documents.nationaldb.org/DeafBlindAssessmentGuide_Rowland.pdf.

Rutter, M., Bailey, A., & Lord, C. (2003a). *Manual for the social communication questionnaire*. Western Psychological Services.

Rutter, M., Le Couteur, A., & Lord, C. (2003b). *Autism diagnostic interview-revised*. Western Psychological Services.

Sampaio, A., Sousa, N., Férnandez, M., Henriques, M., & Gonçalves, O. F. (2008). Memory abilities in Williams syndrome: Dissociation or developmental delay hypothesis? *Brain and Cognition, 66*(3), 290–297. https://doi.org/10.1016/j.bandc.2007.09.005

Shaw, T. A., & Porter, M. A. (2013). Emotion recognition and visual-scan paths in fragile X syndrome. *Journal of Autism and Developmental Disorders, 43*(5), 1119–1139. https://doi.org/10.1007/s10803-012-1654-1

Shearer, A. E., Hildebrand, M. S., Schaefer, A. M., & Smith, R. J. (2023). Hereditary hearing loss and deafness overview. In J. Feldman (Ed.), *GeneReviews*. University of Washington.

Shin, M., Siffel, C., & Correa, A. (2010). Survival of children with mosaic Down syndrome. *American Journal of Medical Genetics Part A, 152*, 800–801. https://doi.org/10.1002/ajmg.a.33295

Smith, N., Sheldrick, R. C., & Perrin, E. C. (2012). An abbreviated screening instrument for autism spectrum disorders. *Infant Mental Health Journal, 34*(2), 134–155. https://doi.org/10.1002/imhj.21356

Sparrow, S. S., Cicchetti, D., & Balla, D. A. (2005). *Vineland adaptive behavior scales, second edition (Vineland-II)*. APA PsycTests. https://doi.org/10.1037/t15164-000

Spencer, M. R., & Hedegaard, H. (2020). QuickStats: Rate of unintentional traumatic Brain injury (TBI)–related deaths among persons aged≤ 24 years, by age group—National Vital Statistics System, United States, 1999–2018. Morbidity and Mortality Weekly Report, 69(41), 1525. https://doi.org/10.15585/mmwr.mm6941a5.

Stadskleiv, K. (2020). Cognitive functioning in children with cerebral palsy. *Developmental Medicine and Child Neurology, 62*(3), 283–289. https://doi.org/10.1111/dmcn.14463

Sterling, A. (2018). Grammar in boys with idiopathic autism spectrum disorder and boys with fragile X syndrome plus autism spectrum disorder. *Journal of Speech, Language, and Hearing Research, 61*(4), 857–869. https://doi.org/10.1044/2017_JSLHR-L-17-0248

Stone, W. L., Basit, H., & Los, E. (2017). *Fragile X syndrome*. StatPearls Publishing. Retrieved January 7, 2023 from https://www.ncbi.nlm.nih.gov/books/NBK459243/.

Stone, W., & Ousley, O. Y. (2008). *Screening tool for autism in toddlers and young children (STAT)*. Vanderbilt University.

Strømme, P., Bjørnstad, P. G., & Ramstad, K. (2002). Prevalence estimation of Williams syndrome. *Journal of Child Neurology, 17*(4), 269–271. https://doi.org/10.1177/088307380201700406

Sullivan, K., Hatton, D., Hammer, J., Sideris, J., Hooper, S., Ornstein, P., & Bailey, D., Jr. (2006). ADHD symptoms in children with FXS. *American Journal of Medical Genetics Part A, 140*(21), 2275–2288. https://doi.org/10.1002/ajmg.a.31388

Sybert, V. P. (1998). Cardiovascular malformations and complications in turner syndrome. *Pediatrics (Evanston), 101*(1), E11. https://doi.org/10.1542/peds.101.1.e11

Sybert, V. P., & McCauley, E. (2004). Turner's syndrome. *New England Journal of Medicine, 351*(12), 1227–1238. https://doi.org/10.1056/NEJMra030360

Symons, F. J., Byiers, B. J., Raspa, M., Bishop, E., & Bailey, D. B., Jr. (2010). Self-injurious behavior and fragile X syndrome: Findings from the national fragile X survey. *American Journal on Intellectual and Developmental Disabilities*, *115*(6), 473–481. https://doi.org/10.1352/1944-7558-115.6.473

Symons, F. J., Clark, R. D., Hatton, D. D., Skinner, M., & Bailey, D. B., Jr. (2003). Self-injurious behavior in young boys with fragile X syndrome. *American Journal of Medical Genetics Part A*, *118*(2), 115–121. https://doi.org/10.1002/ajmg.a.10078

Tsiouris, J. A., & Brown, W. T. (2004). Neuropsychiatric symptoms of fragile X syndrome. *CNS Drugs*, *18*(11), 687–703. https://doi.org/10.2165/00023210-200418110-00001

Twilhaar, E. S., Wade, R. M., De Kieviet, J. F., Van Goudoever, J. B., Van Elburg, R. M., & Oosterlaan, J. (2018). Cognitive outcomes of children born extremely or very preterm since the 1990s and associated risk factors: A meta-analysis and meta-regression. *JAMA Pediatrics*, *172*(4), 361–367. https://doi.org/10.1001/jamapediatrics.2017.5323

United Stated Census Bureau. (2018). American Community Survey: Disability characteristics. Retrieved February 7, 2023 from https://data.census.gov/table?q=hearing+impairment&hidePreview=false&tid=ACSST1Y2018.S1810&vintage=2018.

United States Congress, Public Law 94-142, Education for All Handicapped Children Act (November 29, 1975).

United States Department of Education. (2020, October 16). *OSEP fast facts: Children 3 through 5 served under part B, section 619 of the IDEA*. Individuals with Disabilities Education Act. Retrieved August 7, 2023 from https://sites.ed.gov/idea/osep-fast-facts-children-3-5-20.

Wechsler, D. (2012). *The Wechsler preschool and primary scale of intelligence* (4th ed.). The Psychological Corporation.

Wheeler, A. C., Sacco, P., & Cabo, R. (2017). Unmet clinical needs and burden in Angelman syndrome: A review of the literature. *Orphanet Journal of Rare Diseases*, *12*, 164. https://doi.org/10.1186/s13023-017-0716-z

Whitaker, R., & Thomas-Presswood, T. (2017). School psychological evaluation reports for deaf and hard of hearing children: Best practices. *Journal of Social Work in Disability & Rehabilitation*, *16*(3–4), 276–297. https://doi.org/10.1080/1536710X.2017.1372242

White, K. R. (2014). The evolution of EHDI: From concept to standard of care. In L. R. Schmeltz (Ed.), *A resource guide for early hearing detection and intervention* (pp. 1–32). National Center for Hearing Assessment and Management.

Williams, C. A., Driscoll, D. J., & Dagli, A. I. (2010). Clinical and genetic aspects of Angelman syndrome. *Genetics in Medicine*, *12*(7), 385–395. https://doi.org/10.1097/GIM.0b013e3181def138

Winter, E., Caemmerer, J., Trudel, S., deLeyer, J., Bray, M., Dale, B. A., & Kaufman, A. S. (2023). Does degree of prematurity relate to the Bayley-4 scores earned by matched samples of infants and toddlers across the cognitive, language, and motor domain? *Journal of Intelligence*, *11*, 213–235. https://doi.org/10.3390/jintelligence11110213

World Health Organization. (2021). Deafness and hearing loss. Retrieved January 7, 2023 from https://www.who.int/news-room/fact-sheets/detail/deafness-and-hearing-loss.

World Health Organization. (2022). Preterm birth. Retrieved January 7, 2023 from https://www.who.int/news-room/fact-sheets/detail/preterm-birth.

Yin Foo, R., Guppy, M., & Johnston, L. M. (2013). Intelligence assessments for children with cerebral palsy: A systematic review. *Developmental Medicine and Child Neurology*, *55*(10), 911–918. https://doi.org/10.1111/dmcn.12157

Zhang, D., Kaufmann, W. E., Sigafoos, J., Bartl-Pokorny, K. D., Krieber, M., Marschik, P. B., & Einspieler, C. (2017). Parents' initial concerns about the development of their children later diagnosed with fragile X syndrome. *Journal of Intellectual & Developmental Disability*, *42*(2), 114–122. https://doi.org/10.3109/13668250.2016.1228858

Six

ASSESSMENT TO INTERVENTION

Young children with disabilities receive services in a variety of settings including within the home, school, and clinic. Prior to receiving services, a child must be assessed to help determine if and what services are necessary. Therefore, two of the main goals of assessing young children include (1) to determine if a child should receive or is eligible for intervention services and (2) to help inform the intervention team of current functioning to assist in the development and progress monitoring of appropriate goals (Bracken & Theodore, 2020). Previous chapters in this volume discussed many important aspects of testing a young child, with an emphasis on gathering valid data on a child's functional abilities. This chapter focuses on the various interventions available to the young child.

DON'T FORGET 6.1

Goals of the assessment of infants, toddlers, and preschool children include: (1) to determine if a child should receive or is eligible for intervention services and (2) to help inform the intervention team of current functioning to assist in the development and progress monitoring of appropriate goals.

Within this chapter, we provide an overview of special education law as it relates to eligibility and services for infants, toddlers, and preschoolers. The Individuals with Disabilities Education Act (IDEA, 2004) contains provisions of services for infants and toddlers, birth through 3 under Part C, and for preschool children aged 3–5 under Part B. This chapter includes a discussion

Essentials of Assessing Infants, Toddlers, and Preschoolers, First Edition.
Brittany A. Dale, Joseph R. Engler, and Vincent C. Alfonso.
© 2025 John Wiley & Sons, Inc. Published 2025 by John Wiley & Sons, Inc.

of both eligibility and available intervention for these federal services. We begin with a discussion of early intervention (EI) services for infants and toddlers, including how telehealth may enhance service delivery. We then describe the transition to preschool and relevant services under Part B of IDEA, as well as intervention services available under other federal programs (e.g., Head Start and Section 504). We conclude this chapter with a description of various supplemental therapies that young children can receive in the home, school, and clinic settings.

EARLY INTERVENTION

As discussed earlier in this volume, Part C of the IDEA provides states with federal funding to establish EI services for infants and toddlers with developmental delays or who have a diagnosed condition that makes them at risk for developmental delays. Referral for Part C EI services can be practitioner initiated (i.e., pediatrician, primary care doctor, etc.) or family initiated. Most commonly, the primary care physician identifies a need for intervention and refers to the EI provider. Although children do not need to have a diagnosed condition to be referred for EI services, children with Down Syndrome, autism, cerebral palsy, and those born extremely premature are common conditions referred for services. Once the referral has been made and the family consents, the EI providers have 45 days to conduct the appropriate assessment to determine if eligibility standards are met. Working with the family, the providers conduct assessments across the areas of suspected delays culminating in a formal meeting to develop an initial Individualized Family Service Plan (IFSP), if eligible. The IFSP is discussed in more detail in the following section.

States must adhere to the guidelines set forth in the federal legislation; however, they are responsible for developing their own laws and procedures to implement EI services. Under IDEA Part C, an infant or toddler can be eligible for EI services if they have a diagnosed physical or medical condition that has a high probability of resulting in a developmental delay. These include, but are not limited to, chromosomal abnormalities, congenital infections, disorders secondary to exposure to toxic substances, and low birth weight. Barger and colleagues (2019) conducted a comprehensive review of the diagnosed conditions included in the special education laws across the United States and its territories. These researchers compiled a list of 620 unique conditions that infants and toddlers were diagnosed with to qualify them for EI services under

Part C of IDEA. This research highlights the variability within state special education laws. It is important to note, however, that developmental delays are not necessarily inherent in all these conditions, and assessment is imperative to help determine which functional skill deficits are present that could benefit from intervention.

A young child can also qualify for EI services if they exhibit developmental delays in the absence of a diagnosed condition in any of the five domains of development. These developmental domains include physical development (gross and fine motor; vision and hearing), cognitive development, communication development, social and/or emotional development, and adaptive development. Since individual states have developed their own procedures for determining eligibility for EI services, states vary in their eligibility criteria. For instance, Colorado requires a two standard deviation delay in one developmental domain (McManus et al., 2020), whereas Indiana standards include an additional route to the eligibility of a one-and-a-half standard deviation delay in two developmental areas.

DON'T FORGET 6.2 DEFINITION OF "INFANT OR TODDLER WITH A DISABILITY"

An individual under 3 years of age who needs EI services because the individual (1) is experiencing developmental delays, as measured by appropriate diagnostic instruments and procedures in one or more of the areas of cognitive development, physical development, communication development, social or emotional development, and adaptive development; or (2) has a diagnosed physical or mental condition that has a high probability of resulting in developmental delay.

CAUTION 6.1

Be sure to understand your state's specific eligibility criteria for Part C services as these vary.

Individualized Family Service Plan

When delays are present, children from birth through 3 years old could be eligible for intervention services, which are then outlined in an IFSP. Accurate assessment of this age group is vital to ensure these delays are identified and interventions are appropriately developed. Once identified, children and families work with EI professionals to establish an IFSP.

The IFSP focuses on family-professional partnerships and calls for intervention services to occur in the child's natural environment. Natural environments include the child's home, daycare, or clinic settings. According to McManus and colleagues (2020), physical therapy, occupational therapy, speech therapy, and developmental therapy are the most common EI services. As seen in Rapid Reference 6.1, the IFSP can include a wide range of services that meet the child's needs in the areas of physical development, adaptive behavior, cognitive development, communication, and social-emotional development.

Rapid Reference 6.1 Early Intervention Service Areas

- Family training, counseling, and home visits
- Special Instruction
- Speech pathology and audiology services
- Sign language and cued language services
- Occupational therapy
- Physical therapy
- Psychological services
- Service coordination
- Medical services only for diagnostic or evaluation purposes
- Early identification, screening, and assessment services
- Social work services
- Vision services
- Assistive technology devices and services
- Health services necessary to enable the infant or toddler to benefit from the other EI services
- Transportation and related costs that are necessary to enable an infant or toddler and their family to receive another service listed above

According to IDEA, the IFSP contains several required components (see Rapid Reference 6.2). It must include information on the infant or toddler's current functional levels across the various developmental domains as determined by assessment data. It contains family information including the family's resources, priorities, and concerns. Measurable goals are also included in the IFSP. Table 6.1 includes sample IFSP goals. These goals must include procedures to monitor progress and methods for how to determine when modifications or revisions are needed. Of course, the IFSP also lists the specific EI services the infant or toddler and their family need to reach those goals. The chosen services must be supported by research and provided in the child's natural environment. Details about length of service, duration, frequency, and type of service provider are also included. Additional components include listing a service coordinator, providing a description of any additional medical or related services that are needed, and the dates and duration of the services. Finally, the IFSP must include a plan for transitioning from Part C services to the preschool setting under Part B (IDEA, Sec. 303.344, 2017).

≡ Rapid Reference 6.2 Components of the IFSP

- Infant or toddler's current functional level
- Family information including their resources, priorities, and concerns
- Measurable goals
- A list of EI services that the infant or toddler will receive including duration, frequency, and service provider
- Name of a service coordinator
- Plan for transitioning to the preschool setting

Home-Based Services

As required by IDEA, children aged birth to 3 years must receive services in their natural environment. This means that most infants and toddlers receive intervention services in their home environment. According to the Office of Special

DON'T FORGET 6.3

Intervention services listed in the IFSP should be supported by research and provided in the child's natural environment. Natural environments include the child's home and daycare settings.

Education Programs (OSEP), less than 10% of children received Part C intervention services outside of the home setting (i.e., daycare centers or clinics; United States Department of Education, 2020a). Under Part C requirements, each state establishes its own EI program with a coordinator to oversee service delivery. States also create procedures for qualified EI providers to become contracted to deliver services to children and implement interventions in eligible children's homes.

Table 6.1 Example Goals for Individualized Family Service Plan (IFSP)

Goal	In order to…	We will know we are making progress when…	What are the natural environments for this family?	Strategies and activities…
Child will play with a variety of toys.	participate in preschool readiness.	Imitate unfamiliar actions, engage in reciprocal play, increase the problem-solving, engage in pretend play.	In the home.	Modeling, pretend play, imitation song.
Child will use words to communicate.	not have to point to things so his family knows exactly what he wants.	Decrease frustration, build vocabulary, use words to request items, use words to identify objects, make environmental sounds, make animal noises, put two words together, increase imitation of sounds, and interact with peers.	Home.	Books, songs, finger play, high interest toys, imitation games, modeling, pretend play, play with peers, visit at the playground or library with other children.
Child will use words.	Make choices and explain his wants and needs.	Child imitates sounds and words, he produces a variety of vowel and consonants, he produces word shapes (CV, VC, CVC, VCV, CVCV), and he uses words to make requests.	Home and the gym.	Books, songs, and imitation play.

As described later in this chapter, these service providers include occupational therapists (OTs), speech and language pathologists, physical therapists (PTs), and other developmental therapy providers. Depending on the services established in the IFSP, service providers work with families to develop a schedule of weekly, biweekly, monthly, etc. sessions that meet the child's needs. These service providers enter the families' homes at the scheduled time to provide individual services to children. Therapy sessions may include just the therapist and young child, but they can also include siblings as peer models or parents to ensure continuity of treatment once the provider leaves (Nowell et al., 2022). Parents and other family members may receive coaching from intervention specialists to deliver interventions in the home setting. These interventions are implemented within the infant's or toddler's daily routine and are often combined with naturalistic strategies to promote the most organic implementation of interventions. Intervention providers work with the parent or caregiver to determine which skills should be targeted and how data are collected, and they model implementation strategies to provide parents with the knowledge to conduct interventions independently.

Research has established the efficacy of in-home EI services for young children (Bann et al., 2016; Nowell et al., 2022; Schaub et al., 2019; Wergeland et al., 2022). Specifically, parent-implemented interventions can be efficacious for improving developmental skills in infants and toddlers with delays (Nowell et al., 2022). In families with psychosocial risk factors (e.g., single-parent, parental mental illness, etc.), children who receive home-based EI services show greater development in adaptive skills, including self-care skills and fewer problem behaviors compared to those who do not receive interventions (Schaub et al., 2019). Young children with autism also show improvement in adaptive, cognitive, communication, and socialization skills through home-based intervention. A meta-analysis by Wergeland and colleagues (2022) found that children with autism under the age of 5 years improved their developmental skills when intervention was delivered in the home setting at a comparable rate to interventions conducted in a clinic setting. Home-based EI services may be especially beneficial to children of families with low financial resources. Bann and colleagues (2016) found that young children of low-resourced families who received home-based EI services for the first 3 years of life displayed significantly improved Mental Development Index scores on the Bayley Scales of Infant and Toddler Development, Second Edition (Bayley, 1993) compared to children of high resourced families.

Telehealth and Early Intervention Services

Even before the COVID-19 pandemic beginning in 2020, the use of telehealth to provide EI services was gaining popularity. Telehealth refers to the delivery of health-related services by healthcare providers to clients at a distance (Camden & Silva, 2021). Quality EI services are contingent on the availability of trained service providers, and unfortunately, many communities lack access to these quality providers. Specifically, rural communities appear to have the most significant shortages of qualified professionals available to provide services (Cason et al., 2012; Yang et al., 2020). Shortages exist in common services such as speech and language, but many families in more remote locations do not have access to specialists. Use of secured telehealth platforms can increase interprofessional collaboration, and infants and toddlers can benefit from the services of specialists who they would otherwise never see (Cason et al., 2012). Increased flexibility for visits was also seen as a benefit of telehealth as service providers could see more families, offer nontraditional service hours, and visit with families more often (Cole et al., 2019).

Data on the efficacy of EI via telehealth is emerging. Kronberg and colleagues (2021) studied the use of a parent coaching intervention during the early months of the COVID-19 pandemic. They found improved child performance toward their identified goals and greater parent satisfaction with the interventions. Little and colleagues (2018) also found that families of children with autism reported a telehealth intervention program to be effective and acceptable, and they further discovered the potential for cost savings versus a clinic-based or home-based intervention. Telehealth for assessment of developmental disabilities is also gaining acceptance. Families can face long waitlists for comprehensive developmental assessments (Kanne & Sommer, 2021), and telehealth may alleviate the demand and provide more timely access to services. Research shows families approve of telehealth as an appropriate method of assessment for young children with disabilities (Esther et al., 2022). Families find it convenient and time-saving, and clinicians reported better consultation with other service providers and flexibility in scheduling appointments as benefits of teleassessment.

Although telehealth may be a potential solution to reach more infants and toddlers, several barriers exist. For instance, rural families who may benefit the most from telehealth may not have access to a secure internet connection or computer to participate in such services (Cole et al., 2019). Parents reported internet connectivity and problems with audio and technical glitches on the telehealth platform as the most common problems related to technology (Esther et al., 2022). Clinicians report difficulty with the variable attention of young children, which contributes to difficulty obtaining accurate behavioral observation data. Prior to recommending telehealth services for an infant, toddler, or preschool child, practitioners must perform a needs assessment during the initial evaluation. They should determine the feasibility of services with the available technology of the service provider and family, and work with the family to determine if the child's goals can be met with telehealth services. Service providers should also be aware that although telehealth can fill holes in assessment and service delivery, overall, families prefer face-to-face appointments (Esther et al., 2022).

> **DON'T FORGET 6.4**
>
> Examiners, special educators, and other intervention specialists must conduct a family needs assessment at the initial contact to ensure the use of telehealth is feasible for the family.

TRANSITION FROM EI TO PRESCHOOL

The third birthday marks a pivotal transition point where children who received EI services through Part C transition out of the program. The U.S. Department of Education (2020a) reports the most common outcomes for young children during the transition period. These outcomes include enrolling in preschool under Part B eligibility, withdrawal from services by a parent, and completion of IFSP goals prior to maximum age (U.S. Department of Education, 2020a). Ninety days prior to their third birthday, the IFSP team creates a plan for transitioning out of Part C services. If the young child has not met their IFSP goals, the team refers the family to the local school district for an evaluation to determine if the child may now be eligible for services under Part B of IDEA. These children, however, do not automatically qualify for Part B services, an outcome that many parents find difficult to understand. Children must be evaluated in every area of suspected disability by the multidisciplinary team. The potential disability categories were listed in Rapid Reference 1.2 (Chapter 1 of this volume), with the most common being Speech and/or Language Impairment, Developmental Delay, and Autism for preschool children (U.S. Department of Education, 2020b).

Research has identified several barriers for families when going through the transition process. Malone and Gallagher (2009) identified that the transition from Part C services to the school setting at age 3 years was complicated by several factors, including not completing the appropriate assessments for the transition process. Paperwork is often needed to facilitate the transition process and ensuring that all the appropriate paperwork makes it to the school multidisciplinary team in time for the child's third birthday can be difficult. Families may not return all the necessary paperwork or have difficulty obtaining the appropriate medical and residential documents needed for enrollment. The state's EI program might not send their progress notes, IFSPs, and records to the school in time. When multidisciplinary teams have little information about a child, they must adapt and obtain all necessary information on the day of the evaluation. Often, teams have families complete developmental history questionnaires and sign the appropriate consent on the day of the evaluation and must be quick to gather all the appropriate tests.

Additionally, families often struggle with being removed from the intervention process once their child transitions to the preschool setting. When children receive weekly EI services in the home environment, families become integral to service delivery. They also receive consistent feedback on their child's development and progress toward their goals. Upon entry into school, parents and caregivers may feel like they are outsiders in the process and do not perceive direct benefits to the family (Podvey et al., 2013). In other words, the focus shifts from the family during EI to the child during the preschool years. Furthermore, some families find that their child qualified for EI services but are now told that they do not require these services in the school environment (U.S. Department of Education, 2020a). Qualification for services during EI is based on medical and functional needs within the home, whereas the school must show an educational need for services. For instance, a child with a complex medical history may have required physical therapy services during EI to learn to walk. During the transition evaluation, the PT assesses for developmental milestones in gross motor skills. Within the school environment, this would include whether the child can climb stairs, safely navigate playground equipment, and move safely to the school cafeteria. Even if the child shows some delayed skills across the assessment, they may not qualify for school-based services if they can safely navigate the school environment. In this scenario, parents may struggle to accept that much-needed therapy in the home environment was not deemed necessary within the school environment.

PRESCHOOL SERVICES

The majority of IDEA funds are allocated to Part B appropriations for the grants-to-state program and the preschool education program. For states to receive these funds, they must create a system consistent with the federal rules that provides a free and appropriate public education to all students with qualifying disabilities. In 2020, 6.75% of the nation's children ages 3 through 5 years old received special education services under Part B, Section 619 of IDEA (U.S. Department of Education, 2020b). Under Part B, children must meet eligibility criteria for one of 13 disability categories included in IDEA. Once children are found eligible, the majority receive special education services in the local public school district. A smaller number, as described in the following section, receive services through Head Start.

Similar to eligibility for EI services, states must develop their own definitions of the eligibility categories that fit with the federal guidelines to receive these preschool funds; therefore, state definitions of the educational categories vary. Timelines for evaluations also vary. According to IDEA, the evaluation must be completed within 60 days of when the parent signs consent for the evaluation. To comply, states must develop guidelines that fit within this 60-day timeline regardless of whether school or calendar days are used. Additionally, state special education laws define what assessment tools must be included in the evaluation process. The category of autism provides several examples of how states may vary in assessment and eligibility. Some states require that a pediatrician or clinician be included on the multidisciplinary team or provide a medical diagnosis, while others do not require an outside diagnosis (MacFarlane & Kanaya, 2009). Assessment strategies also vary as only 30% of states require autism specific measures (Pennington et al., 2014). As noted earlier, states also vary in their definition of developmental delay with many focusing on the variability of the obtained standard score from the mean (Alfonso et al., 2020; Danaher, 2011). The category of developmental delay is also age dependent. IDEA states that a child aged 3–9 years old through 9 years, or any other variation (e.g., aged 3 through 5 years old) can be considered for services with a developmental delay. This federal definition allows for states to determine the age range of this category (not exceeding age 9 years)

> # CAUTION 6.2
>
> The multidisciplinary team will only have a predetermined amount of time to complete the eligibility evaluation. Schools may be subject to penalties if evaluations are not completed on time.

and assessment specialists should be aware that a large number of children in the school environment will be eligible under this category. They must also make parents aware that reevaluation is vital to determine accurate eligibility categories as the child ages out of the category of developmental delay.

Team-Based Approach

Within the preschool setting, multidisciplinary or interdisciplinary evaluations are common. Interdisciplinary and multidisciplinary approaches differ in the level of collaboration present throughout the evaluation. The multidisciplinary approach involves multiple practitioners independently conducting their own evaluations under their discipline-specific expertise and then consulting with other team members at the end of the evaluation period (Pfeiffer et al., 2019). At the end of the evaluation process, each team member creates their own written report that is shared among the team. Under a multidisciplinary approach, team members might not be aware of others' findings until the IEP team meeting. The multidisciplinary method lacks the coordination with other team members throughout the process. The interdisciplinary model, on the other hand, focuses on a more integrated approach to the assessment. Under this approach, team members collaborate throughout the evaluation process and discuss findings along the way. Although each team member completes their portion of the evaluation, a single integrated evaluation report is written. Within an early childhood setting, the interdisciplinary approach naturally fits with the characteristics of assessing young children that were presented in Chapter 2 of this volume. Whenever possible, practitioners should utilize the assessment methods that allow for the greatest amount of collaboration.

> # DON'T FORGET 6.5
>
> Interdisciplinary and multidisciplinary approaches differ in the level of collaboration present throughout the evaluation.

School psychologists are experts at eligibility and considered as highly influential during IEP team meetings when making eligibility decisions (Sullivan et al., 2019). However, eligibility determination is always made by the IEP team with all members providing input. The IEP team includes the child's parents, a regular education teacher, a special education teacher, a representative or administrator of the school district, a professional to interpret the evaluation results (i.e., school psychologist), any other individuals invited by the parent or school, and the child (when appropriate; see Rapid Reference 6.3). A thorough evaluation of all suspected disability areas must be reviewed at the IEP team meeting so that all members can make informed decisions about eligibility. For instance, the OT will report findings from the fine and perceptual motor and sensory domains, whereas the speech and language pathologist will report assessment results from the communication evaluation. After all pertinent information is presented to the committee, an eligibility determination is made.

≡ Rapid Reference 6.3 IEP Team Members

- The child's parents
- Regular education teacher
- Special education teacher
- Public agency representative
- Evaluation professionals:
    - School psychologist
    - Occupational therapist
    - Speech and language pathologist
    - Physical therapist
- Other individuals invited by parents or school
- The student, when appropriate

Individual Education Program

After a young child is found eligible for preschool services, the IEP team must create the intervention plan (i.e., IEP). As with the IFSP, the IEP has several components that must be addressed. These components include a statement of present levels of functioning, parent concerns, annual goals, progress monitoring, involvement in general education, related services, accommodations, dates, location, and personnel involved in services, and

DON'T FORGET 6.6

INDIVIDUALIZED EDUCATION PROGRAM

A child, ages 3 through 5 years, found eligible for special education services must have an IEP. Per IDEA, the IEP must include (1) the strengths of the child, (2) the concerns of the parents for enhancing the education of their child, (3) the results of the initial evaluation or most recent evaluation of the child, and (4) the academic, developmental, and functional needs of the child.

a transition plan. IDEA mandates parent involvement in the eligibility and program planning process, and parents of young children with disabilities are an integral part of developing the IEP. Parents should have input into all aspects listed in the IEP, especially the strengths and needs of the child and in developing appropriate, meaningful goals. Too often, the multidisciplinary team develops the IEP goals without input from the family, causing them to feel that they are not partners in the process (Kurth et al., 2019). For instance, a special education teacher may come to the IEP team meeting with an already drafted goal that might not match the parent's concerns with the young child's behavior. Instead, special education teachers, speech language pathologists, and related service providers (OTs and PTs) should come to the meeting prepared to discuss the areas of need identified during the evaluation. Then, committee members, in partnership with the family, should develop appropriate goals to meet the current needs of the child. Parent–school connectedness is an important component of parent IEP satisfaction (Kurth et al., 2019; Slade et al., 2018). Additionally, IEPs must be reviewed at least annually by the IEP team, with reassessment occurring at least every 3 years. Parents may request a conference to discuss IEP goals at any time and should be updated periodically on their child's progress.

Goal Setting

Early childhood special educators and the IEP team rely on accurate assessment to assist them with IEP goal development. As noted above, the school psychologist and other assessment professionals (i.e., speech and language pathologist, OT, etc.) present the results of the evaluation during an IEP team meeting. Based on the areas of need, early childhood educators will work with the families and the rest of the team to create appropriate intervention goals. For instance, if a preschool child qualified for the eligibility category of Developmental Delay and presented with deficits in adaptive skills, the IEP team could look to the assessment measure to find areas for intervention. If a parent or teacher endorsed that the child had difficulty taking off their jacket, a multidisciplinary team may create an IEP goal for the child that focuses on successfully engaging in the morning routine by placing their jacket and backpack in their cubby.

IEP goals are often written as SMART goals. SMART stands for specific, measurable, attainable, relevant, and time-bound. Rapid Reference 6.4 describes each of these key features of SMART goals. Appropriate, well-defined

IEP goals not only inform the IEP team and parents but are essential for school administration to display that they are meeting the federal guidelines of IDEA (Hedin & DeSpain, 2018). Table 6.2 includes sample goals for preschool children based on various developmental needs.

≡ Rapid Reference 6.4 Smart Goals

- Specific   Include specific details about what, when, and how the goal will be accomplished.
- Measurable   Must be something where data can be taken and tracked for progress over time.
- Attainable   The goal should be something that the team believes the child can achieve in the given timeframe.
- Relevant   Goals should relate back to the young child's needs as presented by the parents or discovered in the evaluation.
- Time-bound   Determine the timeline for achieving the goal.

Table 6.2 Example Goals for Age-Appropriate Skills in Preschool

Area	Specially Designed Instruction	Goal Statement
Literacy	Teachers will use visual and verbal models to help Child learn letter recognition, direct instruction, and small group instruction centered around literacy, and multisensory teaching strategies to help Child reach this goal.	When given a printed letter and asked, "What letter?" Child will name at least 10 uppercase letters improving reading skills from 0 to identifying 10 uppercase letters across 4 out of 5 data days as measured by staff observation and data collection.
Numeracy	Teachers will use visual and verbal models to help Child learn rote counting, direct instruction and small group instruction centered around mathematics, and repetition strategies to help Child reach this goal.	When given a verbal request to "count to number 10," Child will rote count to the specified number improving from 2 to numbers up to 10, in 4 out of 5 data opportunities as measured by staff observation, and data collection.

(*Continued*)

Table 6.2 (Continued)

Area	Specially Designed Instruction	Goal Statement
Adaptive Skills	Teachers will use scaffolding and fading support with Child to complete the tasks independently. Verbal and visual prompts will be given, with fading support to help Child gain independence with this goal.	When given an assigned structured activity, Child will work independently at the task for at least 10 minutes with no adult prompts in 4 out of 5 consecutive opportunities as measured by staff observation and data collection.
Following Directions	Specially designed instruction may include but is not limited to the following: adult modeling, visual/pictures, verbal cues and direct instruction to assist in achieving this goal.	During structured tasks, Child will follow 1–2 step directions with embedded basic concepts with 70% accuracy independently across 2 data collection sessions.
Language	Modeling, visual/pictures, verbal cues. and direct instruction will be used to assist in achieving this goal.	When commenting, Child will use a 4+ word sentence at 80% during two sessions.
Color Identification	Teachers will use visual and verbal models to help Child learn the 11 basic colors, direct instruction, and small group instruction centered around mathematics, and repetition strategies to help Child reach this goal.	During a structured task, Child will match 11 basic colors with 80% accuracy on 4 out of 5 data collection opportunities.
Play	Teachers will use modeling and fading support Child to exhibit appropriate functional play. Verbal and visual prompts will be given, with fading support to help Child gain independence with this goal.	When given an opportunity to play, Child will independently exhibit appropriate functional play, for at least 5 minutes over 3 data collections as measured by staff observation.
Receptive Vocabulary	Specially designed instruction may include adult modeling, visual/ pictures, verbal cues, and direct instruction to help achieve this goal.	When presented with objects or pictures placed in a receptive field of 3, Child will point to the verbally prompted object/ pictures with 70% accuracy independently in 2 out of 3 data collection sessions.

Head Start

As discussed in earlier chapters, Head Start and Early Head Start are federally funded early childhood programs designed to provide quality instruction to low-income children. These programs promote school readiness for children under the age of five and focus on building skills across the developmental domains. According to the United States Department of Health and Human Services (2015), Head Start Early Learning Outcomes include Approaches to Learning, Social and Emotional Development, Language and Literacy, Cognition, and Perceptual, Motor, and Physical Development. See Rapid Reference 6.5 for examples of these outcome domains. These central domains closely align with the developmental domains that are discussed in IDEA Part C and Part B intervention services for children with delays and pertain to both Head Start and Early Head Start programs.

≡ Rapid Reference 6.5 Head Start Early Learning Outcomes for Infant/Toddlers and Preschoolers

Domain	Definition	Examples
Approaches to Learning	This is how children learn, how they learn new skills and engage in behaviors. This is linked to success in school. This domain captures several domains: emotional, behavioral, and self-regulation.	Developing coping strategies to follow the rules among peers, following multi-step directions, and deciding roles in pretend play.
Social and Emotional Development	Social Development is making and maintaining relationships with others. The level of these relationships impacts the way children interact with their world. Emotional Development is identifying, coping, and expressing emotions and recognizing and responding to others' emotions.	Creating friendships, compromising, sharing, identifying when they feel mad versus happy, and identifying when others feel sad versus excited.

(continued)

≡ *Rapid Reference 6.5*

Domain	Definition	Examples
Language and Literacy	Language development has two parts: receptive (listening to language) and expressive language (speaking). Literacy refers to pre-reading and writing skills.	Listening to others, tell stories, speaking in sentences, responding to what someone else is saying, repeating songs, asking questions about books that are read to them, and knowing letters.
Cognition	Cognitive Development is the testing of the world around them to understand how it works.	Learn what happens when they flip a light switch, engage in pretend play, laugh when others laugh, and repeat patterns from songs.
Perceptual, Motor, and Physical Development	These are senses and abilities to assist children in learning about their environment.	
Perception	The use of senses to take information from the world and respond to it.	Walking carefully on ice, pressing on sand to collapse the sandcastle, and throwing a ball towards someone.
Gross Motor	Moving the large muscles of the body in arms, legs, head, neck, and torso.	Being able to sit or stand, walking, and playing tag.
Fine Motor	Moving the small muscles of the body, such as those in hands, feet, and face.	Using a pencil to draw, eating with a spoon, brushing teeth, and putting beads on string.
Health, Safety, and Nutrition	This is the knowledge of safe behaviors and routines.	Knowing how to use a toothbrush and communicating when they do not feel well.

Source: Adapted from https://eclkc.ohs.acf.hhs.gov/sites/default/files/pdf/elof-ohs-framework.pdf.

According to federal guidelines, at least 10% of the Head Start program enrollment should be children identified with disabilities. When a child attending a Head Start Program is suspected of having a disability, they are referred to the local educational agency (LEA) responsible for implementing services under IDEA (i.e., the local public school). At that point, the multidisciplinary team from the local school system conducts an eligibility evaluation consistent with what is conducted in the public school setting. Once eligibility is established, an IEP is developed by the IEP team and describes the type and location of services. A child with a disability who attends Head Start could receive their intervention services at the Head Start location, or within the public school setting. For instance, a special education teacher, speech pathologist, and OT could travel to the Head Start location one day per week to meet the weekly intervention minutes listed in the child's IEP. In this scenario, the student receives their special education, related therapies, and general preschool curriculum in the same location. An IEP team might also determine that a child's educational goals would best be met with attending the public preschool setting part-time while attending Head Start the rest of the week. Other potential intervention scenarios could include full-time placement at the public preschool, or full-time placement at Head Start with walk-in therapy services (speech, OT, or PT) at the public school.

DON'T FORGET 6.7
HEAD START
10 PERCENT RULE

Ten percent of all children in Head Start Programs are identified with disabilities. This means that school examiners may conduct educational evaluations in multiple settings.

Section 504 of the Rehabilitation Act of 1973

Preschool children ages 3 through 5 who do not qualify for special education services under IDEA may still be found eligible for accommodations under Section 504 of the Rehabilitation Act of 1973, often referred to as simply Section 504. Administered by the Office of Civil Rights, Section 504 prohibits discrimination based on a disability. Children in public preschool, Head Start, and other settings that receive federal funding may be eligible for protection under Section 504. The young child must first be found to have a disability, and it must be determined to limit substantially one of the child's life functions. The definition of disability under Section 504 aligns with IDEA and includes children across the 13 disability categories. A Section 504 plan may be appropriate for a preschool child who is not found eligible for an IEP under IDEA, but still requires services to obtain an appropriate education similar to their peers. In other words, the child requires reasonable modifications and accommodations to receive equal access to education. The difference between Section 504 and an IEP under IDEA comes in the intervention planning phase. Children with a Section 504 plan receive accommodations within their environment to access the general education curriculum, whereas a child with an IEP would receive intervention services to meet their individual goals, which may or may not be at grade level. In other words, if a child requires additional interventions in the school setting, a Section 504 plan may not be enough.

Multi-Tiered Systems of Support in Preschool Settings (MTSS)

With the reauthorization of IDEA in 2004, multitiered systems of support, also referred to as response to intervention/instruction (RTI), became a commonly promoted progress monitoring system for grade-school children. Academic skills are commonly targeted in this model; however, all areas of development can potentially be addressed. In the early education system, MTSS models are becoming increasingly popular to identify young children who might be at risk for disabilities (Carta et al., 2015). The MTSS model includes three tiers of support to catch and intervene with children before they need a referral to special education. The first tier falls under general education, which includes screening measures to ensure children are responding to the instruction. Tier two includes small group instruction, generally conducted by the classroom teacher. In this tier, a teacher may pull aside a small group of children during literacy block and provide additional instruction on the current grade-level standards. Tier three of the model includes individualized, pull-out instruction that might include remedial instruction. See Figure 6.1 for an example of the tiered approach and Alfonso et al. (2020) for additional information on MTSS for preschoolers.

Universal screening of all children in the preschool setting occurs at tier 1. Screenings should target socially relevant skills necessary for success in preschool (Hojnoski & Missall, 2020). As described more thoroughly in Chapter 4 of this volume, kindergarten readiness is considered an important outcome of early childhood education and includes pre-literacy, per-numeracy, and social-emotional skills (Curby et al., 2017; Hustedt et al., 2018;

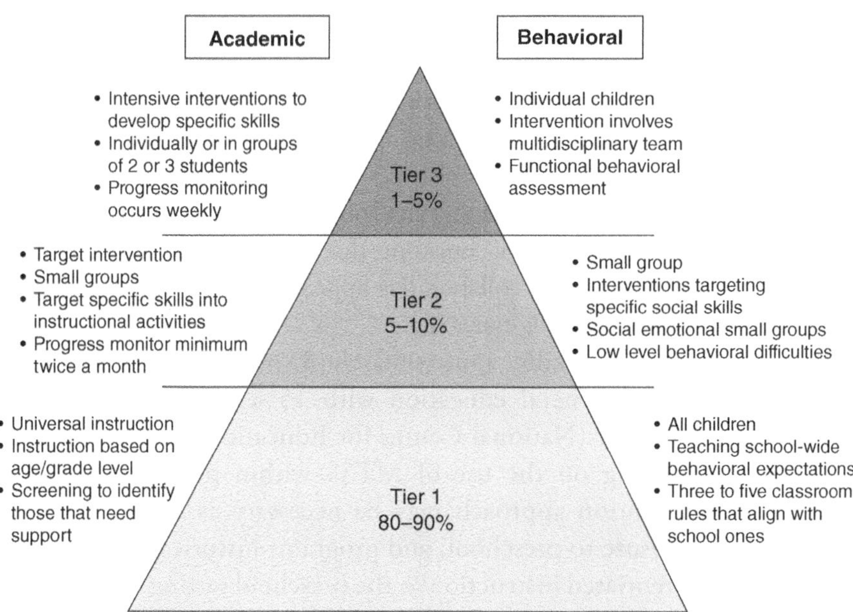

Figure 6.1 Multitier System of Support for Preschoolers *Sources:* **Created using information from Steed and Shapland (2020) and Pierce and Bruns (2013).**

Lin et al., 2020). Teachers complete norm-referenced, standardized rating scales of social-emotional skills for each child, and children participate in quarterly academic assessments completed by teachers. Children who perform below expectations or are flagged for behavioral concerns may be referred for intervention at the higher tiers. Once small-group or individual-tiered interventions begin, progress monitoring must occur to determine if the children are benefitting from the additional instruction. See Chapter 3 of this volume for more information on progress monitoring.

Positive behavior supports (PBS) are commonly employed as a school-wide or class-wide tier I intervention to help improve social outcomes in schools (Barnett et al., 2007). At this initial level, children are exposed to a standard social-emotional curriculum following a research-supported framework (Jones & Bouffard, 2012; Oliver & Berger, 2020). Specifically, the Collaborative for Academic, Social, and Emotional Learning (CASEL, 2013) model stresses the development of self-awareness, social awareness, self-management, relationship skills, and responsible decision-making through structured classroom programming (Engler et al., 2020). A recent meta-analysis indicated positive outcomes for PBS in preschool settings (Luo et al., 2022).

Specifically, children's social and emotional competence increased while challenging behaviors in the classroom decreased. Interventions conducted by personnel other than the classroom teacher and interventions with greater school-family collaboration had more positive outcomes in decreasing challenging behaviors in the classroom. Given that many preschool teachers may lack specific training in managing challenging behaviors in the classroom and may have a high rate of burnout due to classroom-related stress (Raver et al., 2009), taking a collaborative approach to the implementation of PBS in preschool settings is essential.

Regrading academic skills, approximately 85% of grade school aged children respond to general education with 15% of children needing more targeted support (National Center for Education Statistics, 2022). Research is emerging on the use of MTSS within preschool settings. A targeted intervention approach may be necessary as not all children benefit from exposure to preschool, and programs historically struggle to implement differentiated instruction in the preschool setting (Greenwood et al., 2012). Evidence suggests more children in publicly funded early childhood settings may require targeted interventions at the higher tiers, whereas less than 10% of those in tuition-based programs moved up the tiers (Carta et al., 2015).

SPECIALTY SERVICES

As described throughout the sections above, young children can receive many types of necessary therapies through EI and preschool programs. These may include occupational therapy, speech and language therapy, psychological counseling services, physical therapy, and medical services, among others. Along with the school and home settings, young children may also receive these therapies through outpatient clinics. Outpatient intervention services are based on the child's individual needs and can be funded through a family's insurance benefits or they may be an out-of-pocket expense. When recommending supplemental services, examiners should be aware that extra services outside of the federally mandated programs may be a financial burden (Graaf et al., 2022; Vohra et al., 2014). The sections below include summaries of some of the supplemental therapies that are provided across the various settings of in-home, in-school, and outpatient. Some of the differences between settings are highlighted, but a comprehensive review of therapies is beyond the scope of this chapter. See Frolek and Kingsley (2020),

Kennedy and Effgen (2016), Dannemiller and colleagues (2020), and Wergeland and colleagues (2022) for more comprehensive reviews of these supplemental therapies.

Occupational and Physical Therapies

A young child's physical abilities enhance the way in which they explore their world, and a greater capacity to explore leads to greater global skill development (Lobo et al., 2013). PTs and OTs have expert knowledge in the musculoskeletal system, neuromuscular system, and cardiovascular system, and can support the interdisciplinary team as interventions are planned. OTs and PTs often work collaboratively across settings to determine a comprehensive picture of the young child's gross and fine motor skills. Characteristics of these skills and their corresponding assessments were described in Chapter 4 of this volume, and OTs and PTs use the results of these specialized assessments to design appropriate treatment strategies and goals. OTs and PTs can also utilize comprehensive developmental tests, such as the Bayley-4, to assess for motor delays in young children. Research supports the efficacy of motor therapy services for the improvement of skills of young children with developmental delays (Lin & Cherng, 2019). Additionally, early motor intervention has been associated with higher academic skills at kindergarten compared to those who receive delayed intervention (Litt et al., 2017), supporting the longer-term benefits of early motor interventions.

According to the American Occupational Therapy Association, occupational therapy refers to a therapeutic service to support the occupational performance of an individual. For very young children, this includes the occupations of play, eating, moving, dressing, and social interactions (Frolek & Kingsley, 2020). Furthermore, this includes factors that affect an individual's ability to engage in daily living activities, participate in education and work, engage in leisure activities, rest and sleep, and participate in social activities. Children birth to 5 years old receive occupational therapy services for a variety of reasons, including feeding issues, sensory needs, and fine motor delays.

A child would qualify for EI or preschool occupational therapy services if they present with delays based on fine and perceptual motor assessments, sensory processing assessments, or through observed delays based on an OT's expertise (Frolek & Kingsley, 2020). An OT in the schools must answer the question, "How does a delay in this area affect the child's functioning within the preschool classroom?" whereas an outpatient occupational therapy must determine if treatment is medically necessary or falling within the generally accepted standard of care. In other words, OTs (and PTs) must not only determine if there is a delay, but they must also present evidence that the motor delay impacts the child in the preschool classroom (Frolek & Kingsley, 2020).

Speech and Language Therapy

As described in Chapter 4 of this volume, speech and language are distinct categories of communication. A speech and language therapist (SLP) is the primary assessment and service provider for infants, toddlers, and preschool children who exhibit delays in communication. Speech Therapy refers to services that assist children with speaking and articulation. This includes problems with pronunciation, production of sounds, and fluency.

According to OSEP, speech or language impairment makes up the largest category of educational eligibility for children aged 3 through 5 (United States Department of Education, 2020b); therefore, SLPs are indispensable members of the multidisciplinary team. Speech therapy services within the school setting could occur through push-in methods where the SLP enters the child's classroom and elicits the assistance of other children to promote reciprocal communication. These strategies are especially helpful when assessments reveal delays in pragmatic language skills. This strategy would not be available within the outpatient setting and social language skills would need to be practiced with less-than-ideal participants (i.e., adults). Individualized practice of specific speech sounds often happens in a pull-out approach within a preschool. The outpatient clinic provides an ideal setting for these more individualized services within speech therapy. Research suggests parents expect SLPs to conduct individualized treatment in clinic settings without much engagement from the parents during the appointments (Skeat & Roddam, 2019). Parents, however, want guidance about how they can implement strategies that were introduced in the session at home.

Developmental Intervention

As noted above, children who qualify for state-funded EI may be able to utilize services that fall under the category of Special Instruction, which refers to general methods to promote development across all five developmental domains (cognitive, physical, communication, social/emotional, and adaptive). These types of interventions appear to fulfill a vital need for services when a shortage of specialized service providers exists (Cason et al., 2012; Yang et al., 2020). For instance, infants and toddlers in rural areas might qualify for speech and language therapy but may face a shortage of SLPs; therefore, they are placed on waitlist for these services. As a supplemental therapy that can address cognitive, social interaction, and social behavior needs, a developmental therapist can provide intervention to increase communication skills. In this manner, the young child can benefit from some intervention services while waiting for specialized service providers to become available. Special instruction services may also include parent support services through parent education so that enhancement of developmental skills can occur beyond therapist visits.

Behavioral Therapy

Applied behavior analysis (ABA) therapy is an efficacious therapy for children with neurodevelopmental disabilities, including autism spectrum disorder (ASD). Although it is not exclusively utilized with children with ASD, ABA is a highly sought-after treatment for young children with ASD. Research indicates improvement in the cognitive, communication, motor, social-emotional, and adaptive skills of toddlers diagnosed with ASD, and these toddlers displayed greater gains in adaptive and communication skills when intervention began at an earlier age (i.e., younger than 27 months; Vietze & Lax, 2020).

Based on the behavioral principles of B. F. Skinner, ABA began to grow as a science in the 1960s with the application of Skinner's work to human subjects (Wolf et al., 1964). Wolf and colleagues utilized operant conditioning principles to reduce the negative behaviors of a 3.5-year-old child with autism. Using various reinforcers, including food, researchers were able to show a reduction in the child's temper tantrums, increased use of glasses, and a decrease in sleeping problems. Ivar Lovass furthered this science by developing an intensive intervention program for autistic children, which included up to 40 hours of weekly behavior intervention. His intervention program produced positive increases in measured IQ for young children (less than 48 months) with ASD when participating in intensive behavioral therapy (Lovaas, 1987). Today, ABA therapy is one of the most researched forms of treatment for young children with autism and other behavioral disorders.

When a young child receives behavioral therapy, a behavior intervention plan (BIP) is often used to create goals and monitor the young child's progress toward those goals. These plans can be developed through the process of a functional behavior assessments (FBA), which are completed by a clinic-based or educational team. The goal of an FBA is to identify why a child is engaging in a challenging behavior by hypothesizing the function that maintains the behavior (Sam & AFIRM Team, 2022). Rapid Reference 6.6 summarizes the steps of the FBA process. The FBA uses both direct and indirect measures of a child's behaviors (Alter et al., 2008). Direct measures include observation worksheets that code the occurrence of the antecedents, behaviors, and consequences of the child within the natural setting. Indirect measures, on the other hand, include interviews, questionnaires, records reviews, and rating scales completed by parents, teachers, and other caregivers who have intimate knowledge of the young child. The behavioral team members work together to collect and analyze the data, ultimately leading to an intervention plan designed to minimize challenging behaviors and increase positive replacement behaviors.

≡ Rapid Reference 6.6 Steps in the Functional Behavior Assessment Process

1. Establish a multidisciplinary team
2. Identify and define interfering behavior
3. Review records of learner
4. Select assessment procedures
5. Develop plan for collecting data
6. Collect data using selected assessment procedures
7. Collect data on the occurrence of the interfering behavior
8. Analyze collected data
9. Develop a hypothesis statement
10. Test the hypothesis to ensure it is correct
11. Identify appropriate EBPs to address the interfering behavior
12. Develop the behavior intervention plan
13. Monitor the progress of the plan
14. Make changes to the plan as needed

Source: Adapted from https://afirm.fpg.unc.edu/functional-behavior-assessment.

SUMMARY

Evaluations of young children aim to identify if functional deficits are present, which could lead to eligibility for various types of interventions as part of a free and appropriate education. This chapter summarized the various types of interventions that young children with disabilities could benefit from, especially those that fall under federal education law (e.g., IDEA, Section 504, and Head Start and Early Head Start). Examiners first determine if a young child is eligible for intervention services through the various developmental assessments described in Chapter 4. Infants and toddlers from birth to 36 months who have conditions that make them at risk for disabilities or who display delays in any of the five developmental domains (e.g., cognitive, physical, adaptive, communication, and social-emotional) can be eligible for EI services under Part C of IDEA. Preschool-aged children (3 through 5 years) can be eligible for school-based intervention services if they qualify as a child with a disability in one of the 13 categories of IDEA. Various types of intervention services were described with an emphasis on how accurate assessment leads to the development of appropriate goals in these areas.

TEST YOURSELF

1. **The goal of assessing infants, toddlers, and preschoolers is to:**
    (a) To determine if a child should receive or is eligible for intervention services
    (b) To help inform the intervention team of current functioning to help develop and monitor appropriate goals
    (c) A and B
    (d) Neither A nor B

2. **Who can initiate a referral for Part C early intervention services:**
    (a) Primary care doctor
    (b) Family member such as the parent
    (c) Pediatrician
    (d) All the above

3. **How many days do early intervention (EI) providers have to conduct an evaluation to determine if they are eligible for services:**
    (a) 45
    (b) 50

(c) 75

(d) 90

4. Which of the following is/are Early Intervention Service Area(s):

(a) Psychological services

(b) Occupational therapy

(c) Transportation

(d) All the above

5. Which of the following is not a component of an Individualized Family Service Plan (IFSP):

(a) Measurable goals

(b) Functional level across domains

(c) Family information (i.e., resources, priorities, and concerns)

(d) Ability to function in academic settings

6. Research indicates parent implemented interventions can be efficacious for improving developmental skills in infants and toddlers with delays.

(a) True

(b) False

7. Telehealth has the following benefits:

(a) Families find it convenient

(b) It is time saving

(c) Increased flexibility in scheduling and increased consultation

(d) All the above

8. Which of the following is a reported limitation of telehealth:

(a) Low access to secure internet

(b) Practitioner is not able to see the child in the sessions

(c) Parents do not complete the interventions with fidelity

(d) None of the above

9. Which approach involves multiple practitioners independently conducting their own evaluations under their discipline-specific expertise and then consulting with other team members at the end of the evaluation period:

(a) interdisciplinary

(b) multidisciplinary

(c) A and B

(d) Neither A nor B

10. When making goals, the acronym SMART stands for:

(a) Specific, maintained, attainable, reasonable, and time-bound

(b) Studious, maintained, attainable, reasonable, and time-bound

(c) Specific, measurable, attainable, relevant, and time-bound

(d) Similar, measurable, attainable, repetition, and time-bound

Answers: 1. c; 2. d; 3. a; 4. d; 5. d; 6. a; 7. d; 8. a; 9. b; 10. c

REFERENCES

Alfonso, V. C., Ruby, S., Wissel, A. M., & Davari, J. (2020). School psychologists in early childhood settings. In F. C. Worrell & T. L. Hughes (Eds.), *The Cambridge handbook of applied school psychology* (pp. 579–597). Cambridge University Press.

Alter, P. J., Conroy, M. A., Mancil, G. R., & Haydon, T. (2008). A comparison of functional behavior assessment methodologies with young children: Descriptive methods and functional analysis. *Journal of Behavioral Education, 17*, 200–219. https://doi.org/10.1007/s10864-008-9064-3

Bann, C. M., Wallander, J. L., Do, B., Thorsten, V., Pasha, O., Biasini, F. J., Bellad, R., Goudar, S., Comba, E., McClure, E., & Carlo, W. A. (2016). Home-based early intervention and the influence of family resources on cognitive development. *Pediatrics, 137*. https://doi.org/10.1542/peds.2015-3766

Barger, B., Squires, J., Greer, M., Noyes-Grosser, D., Martine Eile, J., Rice, C., Shaw, E., Surprenant, S., Twombly, E., London, S., Zubler, J., & Wolf, R. B. (2019). State variability in diagnosed conditions for IDEA part C eligibility. *Infants & Young Children, 32*(4), 231–244. https://doi.org/10.1097/IYC.0000000000000151

Barnett, D. W., VanDerHeyden, A. M., & Witt, J. C. (2007). Achieving science-based practice through response to intervention: What it might look like in preschools. *Journal of Educational and Psychological Consultation, 17*, 31–54. https://doi.org/10.1207/s1532768Xjepc1701_2

Bayley, N. (1993). *Bayley scales of infant and toddler development—Second edition.* The Psychological Corporation.

Bracken, B. A., & Theodore, A. A. (2020). Observation of preschool children's assessment-related behaviors. In V. C. Alfonso, B. A. Bracken, & R. J. Nagle (Eds.), *Psychoeducational assessment of preschool children* (5th ed., pp. 32–54). Routledge.

Camden, C., & Silva, M. (2021). Pediatric telehealth: Opportunities created by the COVID-19 and suggestions to sustain its use to support families of children disabilities. *Physical & Occupational Therapy in Pediatrics, 41*(1), 1–17. https://doi.org/10.1080/01942638.2020.1825032

Carta, J. J., Greenwood, C. R., Atwater, J., McConnell, S. R., Goldstein, H., & Kaminski, R. A. (2015). Identifying preschool children for higher tiers of language and early literacy instruction within a response to intervention framework. *Journal of Early Intervention, 36*(4), 281–291. https://doi.org/10.1177/1053815115579937

Cason, J., Behl, D., & Ringwalt, S. (2012). Overview of states' use of telehealth for the delivery of early intervention (IDEA Part C) services. *International Journal of Telerehabilitation, 4*(2), 39–46. https://doi.org/10.5195/ijt.2012.6105

Cole, B., Pickard, K., & Stredler-Brown, A. (2019). Report on the use of telehealth in early intervention in Colorado: Strengths and challenges with telehealth as a service delivery method. *International Journal of Telerehabilitation, 11*(1), 33–40. https://doi.org/10.5195/ijt.2019.6273

Collaborative for Academic, Social, and Emotional Learning. (2013). *CASEL schoolkit: A guide for implementing schoolwide academic, social, and emotional learning.* Author.

Curby, T. W., Berke, E., Alfonso, V. C., Blake, J. J., DeMarie, D., DuPaul, G. J., Flores, R., Hess, R. S., Howard, K. A. S., Lepore, J. C. C., & Subotnik, R. F. (2017). Kindergarten teacher perceptions of kindergarten readiness: The importance of social-emotional skills. *Perspectives on Early Childhood Psychology and Education, 2,* 117–137.

Danaher, J. (2011). Eligibility and policies and practice for young children under part B of IDEA. Retrieved June 6, 2023 from http://ectacenter.org/~pdfs/pubs/nnotes27.pdf.

Dannemiller, L., Mueller, M., Leitner, A., Iverson, E., & Kaplan, S. L. (2020). Physical therapy management of children with developmental coordination disorder: An evidence-based clinical practice guideline from the Academy of Pediatric Physical Therapy of the American Physical Therapy Association. *Pediatric Physical Therapy, 32,* 278–313. https://doi.org/10.1097/PEP.0000000000000753

Engler, J. R., Alfonso, V. C., White, J. M., & Ray, C. D. (2020). Assessing social-emotional abilities of preschool-aged children within a social-emotional learning framework. *Perspectives on Early Childhood Psychology and Education, 5,* 171–197.

Esther, C., Natalie, O., Diana, B., Antoinette, H. M., Suzi, D., Marcia, W., & Natalie, S. (2022). Telehealth in a pediatric developmental metropolitan assessment clinic: Perspectives and experiences of families and clinicians. *Health Expectations, 25,* 2557–2569. https://doi.org/10.1111/hex.13582

Frolek, C. G., & Kingsley, K. L. (2020). Practice guidelines—Occupational therapy practice guidelines for early childhood: Birth—5 years. *American Journal of Occupational Therapy, 74,* 1–42. https://doi.org/10.5014/ajot.2020.743001

Graaf, G., Baiden, P., Keyes, L., & Boyd, G. (2022). Barriers to mental health services for parents and siblings of children with special health care needs. *Journal of Child and Family Studies, 31,* 881–895. https://doi.org/10.1007/s10826-022-02228-x

Greenwood, C. R., Carta, J. J., Atwater, J., Goldstein, H., Kaminski, R., & McConnell, S. (2012). Is a response to intervention (RTI) approach to preschool language and early literacy instruction needed? *Topics in Early Childhood Special Education, 33*(1), 48–64. https://doi.org/10.1177/0271121412455438

Hedin, L., & DeSpain, S. (2018). SMART or Not? Writing specific, measurable IEP goals. *Teaching Exceptional Children, 51*(2), 100–110. https://doi.org/10.1177/0040099918802587

Hojnoski, R. L., & Missall, K. M. (2020). Using a multiple-gate assessment approach to support social-emotional development. In M. McLean, R. Banerjee, J. Squires, & K. Hebbeler (Eds.), *Assessment: Recommended practices for young children and families* (pp. 15–24). Division for Early Childhood.

Hustedt, J. T., Buell, M. J., Hallam, R. A., & Pinder, W. M. (2018). While kindergarten has changed, some beliefs stay the same: Kindergarten teachers' beliefs about readiness. *Journal of Research in Childhood Education, 32*(1), 52–66. https://doi.org/10.1080/02568543.2017.1393031

IDEA. (2004). Individuals with Disabilities Education Improvement Act [IDEA] of 2004, 20 U.S.C 1400 et seq.

Jones, S. M., & Bouffard, S. M. (2012). Social and emotional learning in schools: From programs to strategies. *Social Policy Report, 26*(4), 1–33. https://doi.org/10.1002/j.2379-3988.2012.tb00073.x

Kanne, S. M., & Sommer, B. (2021). Editorial perspective: The autism wait-list crisis and remembering what families need. *Journal of Child Psychology and Psychiatry, 62*(2), 140–143. https://doi.org/10.1111/jcpp.13254

Kennedy, E. T., & Effgen, S. K. (2016). Role of physical therapy within the context of early childhood special education. In B. Reichow, B. A. Boyd, E. E. Barton, & S. L. Odom (Eds.), *Handbook of early childhood special education* (pp. 403–417). Springer.

Kronberg, J., Tierney, E., Wallisch, A., & Little, L. M. (2021). Early intervention service delivery via telehealth during COVID-19: A research-practice partnership. *International Journal of Telerehabilitation, 13*(1), 1–8. https://doi.org/10.5195/ijt.2021.6363

Kurth, J. A., McQueston, J. A., Ruppar, A. L., Towes, S. G., Johnston, R., & McCabe, K. M. (2019). A description of parent input in IEP development through analysis of IEP documents. *Intellectual and Developmental Disabilities, 57*, 485–498. https://doi.org/10.1352/1934-9556-57.6.485

Lin, L., & Cherng, R. (2019). Outcomes of utilizing early intervention services on the motor development of children with undefined developmental delay. *Journal of Occupational Therapy, Schools & Early Intervention, 12*, 157–169. https://doi.org/10.1080/19411243.2018.1512437

Lin, L., Tu, Y., Yu, W., Ho, M., & Wu, P. (2020). Investigation of fine motor performance in children younger than 36-month-old using PDMS-2 and Bayley-III. *European Journal of Developmental Psychology, 17*(5), 746–760. https://doi.org/10.1080/17405629.2020.1732917

Litt, J. S., Glymour, M. M., Hauser-Cram, P., Hehir, T., & McCormoick, M. C. (2017). Early intervention services improve school-age functional outcome among neonatal intensive care unit graduates. *Academic Pediatrics, 18*, 468–474. https://doi.org/10.1016/j.acap.2017.07.011

Little, L. M., Wallisch, A., Pope, E., & Dunn, W. (2018). Acceptability and cost comparison of a telehealth intervention for families of children with autism. *Infants & Young Children, 31*(4), 275–286. https://doi.org/10.1097/IYC.0000000000000126

Lobo, M. A., Kokkoni, E., de Campos, A. C., & Galloway, J. C. (2013). Grounding early intervention: Physical therapy cannot just be about motor skills anymore. *Physical Therapy, 93*, 94–103. https://doi.org/10.2522/ptj.20120158

Lovaas, O. I. (1987). Behavioral treatment and normal educational and intellectual functioning in young autistic children. *Journal of Consulting and Clinical Psychology, 55*, 3–9. https://doi.org/10.1037//0022-006x.55.1.3

Luo, L., Reichow, B., Snyder, P., Harrington, J., & Polignano, J. (2022). Systematic review and meta-analysis of classroom-wide social-emotional intervention for preschool children. *Topics in Early Childhood Education, 42*, 4–19. https://doi.org/10.1177/0271121420935579

MacFarlane, J. R., & Kanaya, T. (2009). What does it mean to be autistic? Inter-state variation in special education criteria for autism services. *Journal of Child and Family Studies, 18*, 662–669. https://doi.org/10.1007/s10826-009-9268-8

Malone, D. G., & Gallagher, P. (2009). Transition to preschool special education: A review of literature. *Early Education and Development, 20*, 584–602. https://doi.org/10.1080/10409280802356646

McManus, B. M., Richardson, Z., Schenkman, M., Murphy, N. J., Everhart, R. M., Hambidge, S., & Morrato, E. (2020). Child characteristics and early intervention referral and receipt of services: A retrospective cohort study. *BMC Pediatrics, 20*(84), 1–10. https://doi.org/10.1186/s12887-020-1965-x

National Center for Education Statistics. (2022). Students with disabilities. *Condition of Education.* U.S. Department of Education, Institute of Education Sciences/Retrieved March 16, 2023, from https://nces.ed.gov/programs/coe/indicator/cgg.

Nowell, S., Sam, A., Waters, V., Dees, R., Amsbary, J., & AFRIM Team. (2022). *Parent-implemented intervention for toddlers in the home setting.* The University of

North Carolina at Chapel Hill, Frank Porter Graham Child Development Institute, Autism Focused Interventions Modules and Resources. Retrieved June 6, 2023 from https://afirm/fpg.unc.edu/pii-toddlers.

Oliver, B. M., & Berger, C. T. (2020). Indiana social-emotional learning competencies: A neurodevelopmental, culturally responsive framework. *Professional School Counseling, 23*(1), 1–10. https://doi.org/10.1177/2156759X20904486

Pennington, M. L., Cullinan, D., & Southern, L. B. (2014). Defining autism: Variability in state education agency definitions of and evaluation for autism spectrum disorders. *Autism Research and Treatment, 1–8.* https://doi.org/10.1155/2014327271

Pfeiffer, D. L., Pavelko, S. L., Hahs-Vaughn, D. L., & Dudding, C. C. (2019). A national survey of speech-language pathologists' engagement in interprofessional collaborative practice in schools: Identifying predictive factors and barriers to implementation. *Language, Speech, and Hearing Services in Schools, 50*(4), 639–655. https://doi.org/10.1044/2019_LSHSS-18-0100

Pierce, C. D., & Bruns, D. A. (2013). Aligning components of recognition and response and response to intervention to improve transition to primary school. *Early Childhood Education Journal, 41*(5), 347–354.

Podvey, M. C., Hinojosa, J., & Koenig, K. (2013). Reconsidering insider statues for families during the transition from early intervention to preschool special education. *The Journal of Special Education, 46*(4), 211–222. https://doi.org/10.1177/0022466911407074

Raver, C. C., Jones, S. M., Li-Grining, C., Zhai, F., Metzger, M. W., & Solomon, B. (2009). Targeting children's behavior problems in preschool classrooms: A cluster-randomized controlled trial. *Journal of Consulting and Clinical Psychology, 77,* 302–316. https://doi.org/10.1037/a0015302

Sam, A., & AFIRM Team. (2022). *Functional behavior assessment brief packet, updated.* The University of North Carolina at Chapel Hill, Frank Porter Graham Child Development Institute, Autism Focused Intervention Modules and Resources. Retrieved June 6, 2023 from https://afirm.fpg.unc.edu/functional-behavior-assessment.

Schaub, S., Ramseier, E., Neuhauser, A., Burkhardt, S. C. A., & Lanfranchi, A. (2019). Effects of home-based early intervention on child outcomes: A randomized controlled trial of Parents as Teachers in Switzerland. *Early Childhood Research Quarterly, 48,* 173–185. https://doi.org/10.1016/j.ecresq.2019.03.007

Skeat, J., & Roddam, H. (2019). What do parents think about their involvement in speech-language pathology intervention? A qualitative critically appraised topic. *Evidence-Based Communication Assessment and Intervention, 13,* 15–31. https://doi.org/10.1080/17489539.2019.1600293

Slade, N., Eisenhower, A., Carter, A. S., & Blacher, J. (2018). Satisfaction with individualized education programs among parents of young children with ASD. *Exceptional Children, 84*(3), 242–260. https://doi.org/10.1177/0014402917742923

Steed, E. A., & Shapland, D. (2020). Adapting social emotional multi-tiered systems of supports for kindergarten classrooms. *Early Childhood Education Journal, 48*(2), 135–146.

Sullivan, A. L., Sadeh, S., & Houri, A. K. (2019). Are school psychologists' special education eligibility decisions reliable and unbiased?: A multi-study experimental investigation. *Journal of School Psychology, 77,* 90–109. https://doi.org/10.1016/j.jsp.2019.10.006

U.S. Department of Education. (2020a, June 24). *OSEP fast facts: Infants and toddlers with disabilities.* Individuals with Disabilities Act. Retrieved August 7, 2023 from https://sites.ed.gov/idea/osep-fast-facts-infants-and-toddlers-with-disabilities-20/.

U.S. Department of Education. (2020b, October 16). *OSEP fast facts: Children 3 through 5 served under part B, section 619 of the IDEA.* Individuals with Disabilities Education Act. Retrieved August 7, 2023 from https://sites.ed.gov/idea/osep-fast-facts-children-3-5-20.

U.S. Department of Health and Human Services, Administration for Children and Families, & Office of Head Start. (2015). *Head starts early learning outcome framework: Ages birth to five.* Retrieved August 7, 2023 from https://eclkc.ohs.acf.hhs.gov/sites/default/files/pdf/elof-ohs-framework.pdf.

Vietze, P., & Lax, L. E. (2020). Early intervention ABA for toddlers with ASD: Effect of age and amount. *Current Psychology, 39,* 1234–1244. https://doi.org/10.1007/s12144-018-9812-z

Vohra, R., Madhaven, S., & St. Peter, C. (2014). Access to services, quality of care, and family impact for children with autism, other developmental disabilities, and other mental health conditions. *Autism, 18,* 815–826. https://doi.org/10.1177/1362361313512902

Wergeland, G. J. H., Posserud, M., Fjermestad, K., Ujardvik, U., & Ost, L. (2022). Early behavioral interventions for children and adolescents with autism spectrum disorder in routine clinical care: A systematic review and meta-analysis. *Clinical Psychology: Science and Practice, 29,* 400–414. https://doi.org/10.1037/cps0000106

Wolf, M. M., Risley, T., & Mees, H. (1964). Application of operant conditioning procedures to the behaviour problems of an autistic child. *Behaviour Research and Therapy, 1,* 305–312.

Yang, H. W., Burke, M., Isaacs, S., Rios, K., Schraml-Block, K., Aleman-Tovar, J., Tompkins, J., & Swartz, R. (2020). Family perspectives toward using telehealth in early intervention. *Journal of Developmental and Physical Disabilities, 33,* 197–216. https://doi.org/10.1007/s10882-020-09744-y

Seven

FUTURE DIRECTIONS IN ASSESSMENT OF INFANTS, TODDLERS, AND PRESCHOOLERS

This volume provides up-to-date information regarding the current state of assessing infants, toddlers, and preschoolers. We started by overviewing the history of infant, toddler, and preschool assessments. From there, we discussed unique considerations when assessing young children. Then, we discussed considerations, and advancements, within test design that help practitioners make responsible decisions. Next, we highlighted important developmental domains that should be included in a developmental assessment. We followed with a description of low-frequency disorders that examiners will likely experience throughout their professional careers. Next, we examine the linkage between assessment and intervention strategies.

The final chapter in this volume focuses on the future direction of infant, toddler, and preschool assessment and could be the most difficult to write. That is, the discussion of the future of infant, toddler, and preschool assessment involves a prediction as to where the field is heading. Although once thought of as a benign task, the COVID-19 pandemic taught us all to prepare for the unexpected and that nobody truly knows what the future holds. Regardless, there are trends that we have noticed over time in the research and our professional practice that may be helpful to move the field of infant, toddler, and preschool assessment forward and are the focus of this final chapter. The trends fit relatively nicely into three broad categories. The first category includes the advancement of professional associations and organizations. The second category involves the evolution of infant, toddler, and preschool assessment within an advancing service delivery model. The third category

Essentials of Assessing Infants, Toddlers, and Preschoolers, First Edition.
Brittany A. Dale, Joseph R. Engler, and Vincent C. Alfonso.
© 2025 John Wiley & Sons, Inc. Published 2025 by John Wiley & Sons, Inc.

includes graduate preparation and professional development needs to assist practitioners. We discuss each of these categories within the chapter separately. Then, we summarize the most salient future directions in infant, toddler, and preschool assessment.

ADVANCEMENTS IN PROFESSIONAL ASSOCIATIONS AND ORGANIZATIONS

From a historical context, the formalized study of early childhood education is still in its infancy. We remember back when early childhood education was an afterthought of the K-12 educational system and there was a widespread belief that early childhood educators' sole responsibility was to care for the safety of young children rather than teach young children. Fortunately, the formation of professional associations such as the National Association for the Education of Young Children (NAEYC), the National Association of Early Childhood Specialists in State Departments of Education (NAECS/SDE), the Council for Exceptional Children (CEC), the National Association of School Psychologists (NASP), and others have worked tirelessly to promote continually and professionalize the field. Moreover, the NAEYC has spent over 40 years committed to professional preparation (NAEYC, 2019). In addition, over half of the states have specific standards for early childhood that include elements such as outcomes and learning expectations as of the early 2000s (NAEYC & NAECS/SDE, 2002).

Most recently, the NAEYC published a position statement titled *Professional Standards and Competencies for Early Childhood Educators* (2019). Within the position statement, the NAEYC listed six professional standards and competencies. The standards are: (1) child Development and Learning in Context, (2) Family-Teacher Partnerships and Community Connections, (3) Child Observation, Documentation, and Assessment, (4) Developmentally, Culturally, and Linguistically Appropriate Teaching Practices, (5) Knowledge, Application, and Integration of Academic Content in the Early Childhood Curriculum, and (6) Professionalism as an Early Childhood Educator (See Rapid Reference 7.1). Furthermore, the standards have many competencies embedded within that highlight important knowledge and skills necessary to support early childhood development and learning while maintaining high expectations of early childhood educators in general.

≋ Rapid Reference 7.1 Six Professional Standards Provided by NAEYC (2019)

- Child Development and Learning in Context
- Family-Teacher Partnerships and Community Connections
- Child Observation, Documentation, and Assessment
- Developmentally, Culturally, and Linguistically Appropriate Teaching Practices
- Knowledge, Application, and Integration of Academic Content in the Early Childhood Curriculum
- Professionalism as an Early Childhood Educator

While all standards and competencies have relevancy to this volume, perhaps the most important standard to expand upon is Standard 3, which directly relates to the assessment of young children. Standard 3 includes several competencies that each early childhood educator should demonstrate (NAEYC, 2019). The competencies involve understanding formal and informal assessment as well as formative and summative assessment. In addition, early childhood educators should know a multitude of assessment methods. For example, they should be familiar with screening, observations, standardized, and other types of assessment practices. Early childhood educators should be familiar with the ethical and legal responsibilities necessary to use assessments in fair and equitable ways that are designed to promote positive progress and development for young children. Finally, early childhood educators should develop collaborative partnerships with other professionals, as well as families, as it relates to assessment practices. Moreover, early childhood educators should have the skills necessary to conduct and disseminate assessment data to various stakeholders to help meet the needs of young children.

The efforts made by professional associations and organizations to define more thoroughly and advance the early childhood profession are noticeable, commended, and needed. It underscores, however, that early childhood educators prepared to meet the professional standards and competencies set forth by NAEYC (and others) should work in settings and contexts that support and fully utilize the knowledge, skills, and

DON'T FORGET 7.1

The future direction in the assessment of infants, toddlers, and preschoolers should strive to create settings and contexts where professional standards and competencies are easy to deliver.

professional dispositions needed to meet the needs of young children and their families effectively. Therefore, just as the early childhood profession continues to advance, so do the contexts and settings in which these services are delivered.

PRESCHOOL ASSESSMENT WITHIN AN EVOLVING SERVICE DELIVERY MODEL

For those practicing in traditional K-12 settings, the conceptual framework associated with multitiered system of support (MTSS) may not be new. That said, professionals who spend most of their time in preschool settings may be much less aware. Therefore, we provide a basic overview of MTSS and describe why its application in preschool settings is warranted. As introduced in Chapter 6 of this volume, the conceptual framework known as MTSS was developed to support K-12 students. Moreover, as far back as we can remember, K-12 schools have always had difficulty finding ways to support *all* students' academic and behavioral growth. Additionally, those in K-12 schools wanted to shift away from solely identifying problems to a framework of prevention. In essence, educators wanted a way to prevent academic and behavioral difficulties from occurring in the first place. Prevention is critically important, especially as it relates to preschool-aged children because the research shows that preschools are expelled at a rate more than three times as often as K-12 students (Gilliam, 2005).

To prevent academic and behavior challenges from occurring, MTSS assumes that all young children will not respond adequately (e.g., achieve age-related performance expectations) to the content that is delivered (Kong et al., 2021). Therefore, preschools should provide different levels of academic and behavioral support that are needed prior to referring a young child for a comprehensive evaluation. The different levels of support correspond with different tiers within a MTSS framework. Typically, there are three tiers within the majority of MTSS frameworks. Tier 1 includes all children and involves access to evidence-based academic and behavioral programs. It is estimated that approximately 85% of children will respond adequately and demonstrate academic and/or behavioral performance consistent with age and/or grade-level expectations (Stoiber, 2014).

The remaining children (i.e., 10–15%) are identified as needing additional academic and/or behavioral supports to be successful. Further, the remaining 10–15% of children represent Tier 2 and would need more individualized academic and behavioral supports, which would typically be delivered in small groups (Stoiber, 2014). It is estimated that approximately 5% of children receiving Tier 2 interventions would demonstrate performance inconsistent with age and/or grade level expectations and would need more individualized academic and/or behavioral supports (Stoiber, 2014). These young children would represent Tier 3 in an MTSS framework and would likely receive individualized instruction. Additionally, these young children may be referred for a comprehensive psychoeducational evaluation to assist in determining whether they have a disability.

DON'T FORGET 7.2

MTSS is a preventative framework that attempts to match levels of academic and/or behavioral supports with the needs of children.

To apply an MTSS framework in preschool settings, early childhood educators should have proper preparation regarding two assessment-related practices. The two assessment-related practices are universal screening and progress monitoring. Universal screening involves administering a quick, cost-effective assessment to all young children. The results of the universal screening are often compared to a normative sample and identify young children who may need additional academic and/or behavioral supports (i.e., young children who should be moved to Tier 2). As mentioned earlier, the young children who are identified as needing Tier 2 services receive additional academic and/or behavioral supports. Consequently, early childhood educators will need to monitor progress to determine whether they are making academic and/or behavioral gains to close the identified gap from the universal screening. If the gap closes, the young child may be moved back to Tier 1. If the gap continues, or becomes bigger, the young child may move to Tier 3. For a more thorough description of screening and progress monitoring tools, interested readers are encouraged to see Chapter 3 (this volume) and Nagle et al. (2020).

CAUTION 7.1

Screening and progress monitoring are different than diagnostic tools.

The conceptual framework of MTSS provides much intuitive appeal, especially in a preschool setting. First, it is based upon a preventative approach to supporting young children. Second, it provides a structure for meeting young children where they are developmentally and provides evidence-based support to assist in meeting their academic and behavioral needs. Third, MTSS provides a framework that attempts to intervene prior to referring children for a psychoeducational evaluation. The successful implementation of an MTSS framework relies on early childhood educators being properly prepared to universally screen and progress monitor young children's growth. That said, universal screening and progress monitoring fall within NAEYC (2019) Standards and Competencies and represent an advancement in preschool settings that should have a positive impact on early childhood development. Therefore, we see a direct alignment between the advancement in professional standards and the creation of context-based settings that should foster academic and behavioral development of young children.

Telehealth Service Delivery

The COVID-19 pandemic was an unprecedented event that significantly altered the practice of psychology as we know it. Furthermore, the pandemic forced practitioners to adjust the way psychological services were delivered, while receiving little guidance from professional organizations on how to do so (Wright & Raiford, 2021). We remember vividly the challenges that came during this time. From a professional standpoint, practitioners in many states were not allowed to see clients in person due to health risks. Therefore, practitioners had to figure out how to deliver psychological services in a way that minimized disruptions to the continuity of care. Next, the traditional ways in which some psychological services (i.e., tests) were delivered (i.e., face-to-face) were not conducive to delivery via online modalities. For example, tests that used physical manipulatives could not be administered online. Consequently, practitioners struggled to identify whether the benefits of providing psychological services outweighed the risks and uncertainties. Despite such challenges, the COVID-19 pandemic also provided an opportunity for practitioners to find new and innovative ways to deliver psychological services via tele-assessment.

Not new in its inception, the rate of tele-assessment delivery increased significantly during the COVID-19 pandemic (Wagner et al., 2022). Additionally, there have been numerous studies that have shown the positive effects of delivering treatment via technology (Sutherland et al., 2018). As a result, we anticipate the use of technology to deliver psychological assessments and treatment options will increase in the future. In addition to research supporting its use, there are several potential benefits of tele-assessment. For example, the use of tele-assessment allows greater access to professional services, especially for those who live in rural settings. Additionally, the use of tele-assessment may reduce financial and time barriers associated with traveling a long distance to see a provider. Finally, tele-assessment may allow access to a larger network of providers, and it may reduce the amount of time needed to see a provider (See Rapid Reference 7.2).

≋ Rapid Reference 7.2 Potential Benefits of Tele-Assessment

- Greater access to professional services for those in rural settings
- Reduction in travel-related costs
- Access to a larger network of providers
- Reduction in the time to see a provider

While there are several possible benefits to tele-assessment, there are several considerations to keep in mind. First and foremost, practitioners should always adhere to their state laws and regulations. Second, practitioners should be aware of relevant ethical guidelines related to the use of tele-assessment practices. Third, practitioners should follow the recommendations set forth by professional associations and organizations related to tele-assessment practices. Fourth, practitioners should continually monitor and read the latest research regarding the effectiveness of tele-assessment practices (See Rapid Reference 7.3).

≋ Rapid Reference 7.3 Recommendations Prior to Using Tele-Assessment

- Know and follow all applicable state laws and regulations
- Know and consider all relevant ethical guidelines
- Follow guidance provided by professional associations and organizations
- Continually read research on the effectiveness of tele-assessment

We envision that the role of tele-assessment will continue well into the future. Our hope is that our professional fields continue to use tele-assessment for its numerous benefits while minimizing its drawbacks. We also recognize that tele-assessment is a continuous area of study and look forward to seeing its evolution based upon rigorous research and discernment. We recognize that tele-assessment is not for everybody, but it is for somebody. In particular, we look forward to the day when all young children have access to high-quality care and know that tele-assessment will assist us in getting closer to that day.

Thus far, this chapter has focused on the future directions in the assessment of infants, toddlers, and preschoolers and emphasized the critical role that professional associations and organizations play in the development of early childhood educators. Additionally, we highlighted how the expansive role of early childhood educator needs a setting and/or context to implement the role. The next section of this chapter highlights areas that graduate preparation and professional development can support the future of infant, toddler, and preschool assessment.

GRADUATE PREPARATION AND PROFESSIONAL DEVELOPMENT NEEDS

One of the most direct ways in which graduate preparation interacts with infant, toddler, and preschool assessment is through a course or courses related to assessment. The study of assessment has been a professional topic of discussion for decades. Although it was not the primary focus of their research, Copeland and Miller (1985) surveyed practicing school psychologists on what courses were of most importance at the present time, and what courses were most important in the future. Unsurprisingly, the authors found the need for preparation in assessment to be important in the present and future times. What was surprising, however, was that one of the highest identified future needs for school psychologists was the need for preparation, specifically in infant and preschool assessment. Therefore, the need for infant and preschool assessment has been an identified need in graduate preparation programs for nearly 40 years. One area where infant, toddler, and preschool assessment preparation can be taught is in cognitive assessment classes.

> ## DON'T FORGET 7.3
>
> The identified need for graduate preparation in infant and preschool assessment has been around for at least 40 years.

Approximately one year later, Oakland and Zimmerman (1986) conducted a study where they surveyed 49 course instructors who taught cognitive assessment courses at the graduate level. The results of the survey indicated that the Wechsler Scales and Stanford-Binet were the tests taught most frequently and that test administration, test interpretation, test scoring, and test reporting were rated as the most important topics covered in the course. In contrast, the Bayley Scales of Infant Development was frequently not required to be administered in the course and only 4% of instructors rated infant development as being a very important topic to teach. This provides further evidence that although infant and preschool assessment was rated as a future need in graduate preparation, it was not given its due diligence within the premier course on cognitive assessment. It should be noted that these two studies were within a short proximity. Therefore, it may take time before we would expect to see changes in graduate preparation programs.

Approximately 15 years after Copeland and Miller's study, Alfonso et al. (2000) surveyed 97 instructors of cognitive assessment courses. Alfonso and colleagues found that graduate programs were teaching similar theories, tests, interpretations, and public policies as found in Oakland and Zimmerman's study. Regarding preschool assessment, Alfonso and colleagues found that nearly two-thirds of the cognitive courses are also used to teach the assessment of preschoolers, whereas the remaining one-third had an alternative standalone course that focuses on the assessment of preschoolers. Additionally, many programs that did not have a standalone course on the assessment of preschoolers felt that a separate course was necessary. Finally, no program identified that they teach a standalone course on the assessment of infants.

For too long in our profession, the assessment of young children has been seen as a downward extension in assessing school-aged children, which was seen as a downward extension of assessing adults (Alfonso, Ruby, et al., 2020). Therefore, we recommend that graduate preparation programs begin considering early childhood assessment as its own distinct area of study. To prepare practitioners properly to work with young children, they should have the specific training to do so (Nagle, 2007). While a comprehensive discussion of specific trainings is precluded from this chapter due to length, interested readers are encouraged to see Alfonso, Bracken, et al. (2020) for a comprehensive overview. Instead, however, we will focus on two rapidly emerging trends in infant, toddler, and preschool assessment pertinent to graduate preparation and professional development: advancements in intelligence theory and advancements in test design.

Intelligence Theory

Nearly four decades ago, Lidz (1986) wrote an article regarding the future of preschool assessment. In her article, she discussed the need for the professional community to advance the definition of intelligence with special consideration regarding the relationship between intelligence and cultural and cross-cultural tasks. Although we see the advancement of intelligence with an emphasis on cultural and cross-cultural tasks as continuous, we think we are closer than ever to making this a reality. Since the Lidz (1986) manuscript, we have seen continual advancements in Cattel–Horn–Carroll Theory of Cognitive Abilities (CHC Theory) become very nuanced and well defined. A comprehensive review of CHC Theory is precluded from this chapter due to space considerations; however, it is discussed throughout this volume (see Chapters 3 and 4). Interested readers are also encouraged to see McGrew (2023) and Schneider and McGrew (2018) for more information on CHC Theory.

The advancements in CHC Theory can have a direct influence on the future of infant, toddler, and preschool assessment in many ways. First, as CHC Theory definitions of abilities and psychometrics become more refined and precise, we imagine that tests are going to assess the abilities we want to measure more purely. For example, a subtest may measure multiple broad and/or narrow abilities all at the same time. When this happens, and a young child performs poorly on that subtest, it is difficult to decipher what specific ability is likely causing the deficit. In contrast, if a subtest measures one specific ability, we have more confidence in identifying the cause of the deficit. The advancements in CHC Theory, paired with statistical analyses, are helping practitioners parse out specific abilities of deficit and we envision rapid advancement in this area in the future.

If the advancement of CHC Theory allows practitioners to assess purer measures of skills and abilities, we envision significant advancements in the intervention of those abilities as well. For example, if three abilities are measured and a young child demonstrates a deficit, we do not know which of the abilities to intervene upon. In contrast, if we precisely measure one ability (e.g., attentional control), and a young child has deficits in this area, we can then design specific interventions that are tailored to address it. As a result, we envision the future of intelligence theory as helping practitioners more precisely diagnose and treat specific areas of deficit.

Test Design

Test design for young children has been the subject of criticism for decades (see Braken & Walker, 1997; Nagle et al., 2020). One reason for such criticisms is that many tests for young children were developed as downward extensions of tests for school-aged children (Alfonso & Flanagan, 2009). Consequently, tests for young children had several shortcomings. Fortunately, researchers like Alfonso and Flanagan (2009) have worked to develop qualitative and quantitative criteria so that examiners can evaluate tests to ensure they are used for their intended purposes (Engler & Alfonso, 2020). A more thorough review of the important qualitative and quantitative characteristics necessary to design and develop high-quality tests for young children can be found in Rapid Reference 2.4 and Chapter 3 of this volume.

The ability of researchers to identify important qualitative and quantitative characteristics is necessary to advance the quality of test design for young children continually. First, it provides examiners with an awareness of important characteristics needed to evaluate the overall quality of a test. Second, it allows examiners to match better the selection of a test with the referral question(s) at hand. Third, it allows test publishers to use information gained from this writing and subsequent evaluations of tests to inform continually the design and development of newly published tests (See Rapid Reference 7.4).

≡ Rapid Reference 7.4 How the Identification of Qualitative and Quantitative Characteristics Can Advance Test Design

- Provides examiners with an awareness of important characteristics to evaluate
- Allows examiners to match tests with referral questions
- Allows test publishers to design and develop new tests

SUMMARY

In many ways, the future of assessing infants, toddlers, and preschoolers is quite promising. The advancements and advocacy of professional associations and organizations like NAEYC, NAECS/SDE, CEC, NASP, and others have enhanced the profession of early childhood educators. Moreover, professional associations and organizations provide standards for preparation, while keeping the outcomes of young children at the forefront. The advancements in professional preparation, paired with advanced service delivery models (namely MTSS), have created opportunities to match better academic and behavioral supports to young children in ways not previously possible. Consequently, we are working toward a model that focuses more on prevention than it does identification.

While the predominate modality of assessing infants, toddlers, and preschoolers remains via face-to-face interactions, the advancements in our understanding of tele-assessment provide the possibility for increased access to services, especially for young children in rural settings. The study of tele-assessments is not new, but it has been rapidly expanding since the COVID-19 pandemic.

To prepare early childhood educators for a myriad roles, we turn to the importance of graduate education and call out the need to devote more time and emphasis on early childhood assessment methods, tests, and strategies within graduate preparation programs. This was an identified need decades ago and continues to persist. We also recognize that with advancements in society and technology come advancements such as intelligence theory and test design, which directly influence the future of test development and delivery. We highlight the importance of continued professional development as a way for early childhood educators to remain current in their practices, so that they can continue to deliver high-quality supports and service to young children.

🐾 TEST YOURSELF 🐾

1. **Which of the following is a NAEYC Standard for Early Childhood Educators?**

    (a) Family-Teacher Partnerships and Community Connections

    (b) Child Observation, Documentation, and Assessment

    (c) Professionalism as an Early Childhood Educator

    (d) All of the above

2. **Approximately 30% of young children would need Tier 2 support in a MTSS framework.**

    (a) True

    (b) False

3. **All of the following are potential benefits of an MTSS framework except:**

    (a) It is preventative in nature

    (b) It matches the level of supports to the needs of young children

    (c) It monitors the progress of interventions

    (d) It is diagnostic in nature

4. **Tele-assessment practices first began during COVID-19.**

    (a) True

    (b) False

5. **Practitioners considering using tele-assessment should:**

    (a) Fully understand state laws and regulations

    (b) Consult ethical guidelines

    (c) Follow professional association and organization guidelines

    (d) All of the above

6. **Infant and preschool assessment has been a primary focus of graduate preparation for decades.**

    (a) True

    (b) False

7. **In an early study, only 4% of instructors rated infant development as an important topic to teach.**

    (a) True

    (b) False

8. **Over the past several decades, CHC Theory has:**

    (a) Been debunked

    (b) Remained stagnant

    (c) Rapidly advanced

    (d) Morphed into a new theory

9. **Understanding important qualitative and quantitative characteristics should enhance test design.**

    (a) True

    (b) False

10. The future of infant, toddler, and preschool assessment is bright.

(a) True

(b) False

Answers: 1. d; 2. b; 3. d; 4. b; 5. d; 6. b; 7. a; 8. c; 9. a; 10. a

REFERENCES

Alfonso, V. C., Bracken, B. A., & Nagle, R. J. (2020). *Psychoeducational assessment of preschool children* (5th ed.). Routledge.

Alfonso, V. C., & Flanagan, D. P. (2009). Assessment of preschool children: A framework for evaluating the adequacy of the technical characteristics of norm-referenced instruments. In B. Mowder, F. Rubinson, & A. Yasik (Eds.), *Evidence based practice in infant and early childhood psychology* (pp. 129–166). John Wiley & Sons.

Alfonso, V. C., Oakland, T. D., LaRocca, R., & Spanakos, A. (2000). The course on individual cognitive assessment. *School Psychology Review, 29*(1), 52–64.

Alfonso, V. C., Ruby, S., Wissel, A. M., & Davari, J. (2020). School psychologists in early childhood settings. In F. C. Worrell, T. L. Hughes, & D. D. Dixon (Eds.), *The Cambridge handbook of applied school psychology* (pp. 579–597). Cambridge University Press.

Braken, B. A., & Walker, K. C. (1997). The utility of intelligence tests for preschool children. In D. P. Flanagan, J. L. Genshaft, & P. C. Harrison (Eds.), *Contemporary intellectual assessment: Theories, tests, and issues* (pp. 484–502). Guilford.

Copeland, E. P., & Miller, L. F. (1985). Training needs of prospective school psychologists: The practitioners' viewpoint. *Journal of School Psychology, 23*, 247–254.

Engler, J. R., & Alfonso, V. C. (2020). Cognitive assessment of preschool children: A pragmatic review of theoretical, quantitative, and qualitative characteristics. In V. C. Alfonso, B. A. Bracken, & R. J. Nagle (Eds.), *Psychoeducational assessment of preschool children* (5th ed., pp. 226–249). Routledge.

Gilliam, W. S. (2005). *Prekindergartners left behind: Expulsion rates in state prekindergarten systems.* Yale University Child Study Center.

Kong, N. Y., Carta, J. J., & Greenwood, C. R. (2021). Studies in MTSS problem solving: Improving response to a pre-kindergarten supplemental vocabulary intervention. *Topics in Early Childhood Special Education, 41*(2), 86–99. https://doi.org/10.1177/0271121419843995

Lidz, C. S. (1986). Preschool assessment: Where have we been and where are we going? *Special Services in the Schools, 2*, 141–159. https://doi.org/10.1300/J008v02n02_10

McGrew, K. S. (2023). Carroll's three-stratum (3s) cognitive ability theory at 30 years: Impact, 3s-CHC theory classification, structural replication, and cognitive-achievement psychometric network analysis extension. *Journal of Intelligence, 11*(2). https://doi.org/10.3390/jintelligence11020032

Nagle, R. J. (2007). Issues in preschool assessment. In B. A. Braken & R. J. Nagle (Eds.), *Psychoeducational assessment of preschool children* (4th ed., pp. 29–48). Lawrence Erlbaum Associates.

Nagle, R. J., Gagnon, S. G., & Kidder-Ashley, P. (2020). Issues in preschool assessment. In V. C. Alfonso, B. A. Braken, & R. J. Nagle (Eds.), *Psychoeducational assessment of preschool children* (5th ed., pp. 3–31). Routledge.

National Association for the Education of Young Children. (2019). Professional standards and competencies for early childhood educators. Retrieved April 12, 2024, from https://www.naeyc.org/resources/position-statements/professional-standards-competencies.

National Association for the Education of Young Children, & National Association of Early Childhood Specialists in State Departments of Education. (2002). Early learning standards: Creating the conditions for success. Retrieved April 12, 2024, https://www.naeyc.org/sites/default/files/globally-shared/downloads/PDFs/resources/position-statements/position_statement.pdf.

Oakland, T. D., & Zimmerman, S. A. (1986). The course on individual mental assessment: A national survey of course instructors. *Professional School Psychology*, *1*(1), 51–59.

Schneider, W. J., & McGrew, K. S. (2018). The Cattell-Horn-Carroll theory of cognitive abilities. In D. P. Flanagan & E. M. McDonough (Eds.), *Contemporary intellectual assessment: Theories, tests, and issues* (4th ed., pp. 73–163). The Guilford Press.

Stoiber, K. C. (2014). A comprehensive framework for multitiered systems of support in school psychology. In P. L. Harrison & A. Thomas (Eds.), *Best practices in school psychology: Data-based and collaborative decision making* (pp. 41–70). National Association of School Psychologists Publications.

Sutherland, R., Trembath, D., & Roberts, J. (2018). Telehealth and autism: A systematic search and review of the literature. *International Journal of Speech-Language Pathology*, *20*(3), 324–336.

Wagner, L., Weitlauf, A. S., Hine, J., Corona, L. L., Berman, A. F., Nicholson, A., Allen, W., Black, M., & Warren, Z. (2022). Transitioning to telemedicine during COVID-19: Impact of perceptions and use of telemedicine procedures for the diagnosis of autism in toddlers. *Journal of Autism and Developmental Disorders*, *52*, 2247–2257. https://doi.org/10.1007/s10803-021-05112-7

Wright, A. J., & Raiford, S. E. (2021). *Essentials of psychological tele-assessment*. John Wiley & Sons Inc.

APPENDIX: INFANT AND TODDLER ASSESSMENTS BY DOMAIN

Essentials of Assessing Infants, Toddlers, and Preschoolers, First Edition.
Brittany A. Dale, Joseph R. Engler, and Vincent C. Alfonso.
© 2025 John Wiley & Sons, Inc. Published 2025 by John Wiley & Sons, Inc.

SUMMARY OF CURRENT INFANT AND TODDLER ASSESSMENTS

Test Name	Author(s) (Year of Publication)	Age Range	Developmental Domains or Areas Assessed
American Association for Mental Deficiency (AAMD) Adaptive Behavior Scale – Revised (AAMD ABS)	Nihira et al. (1993)	3 years–69 years	Mental, Emotional, and Developmental Disabilities
AAMD Adaptive Behavior Scale – School Edition (ABS-SE)	Lambert and Windmiller (1981)	3 years 3 months–17 years 2 months	Mental, Emotional, Adaptive Behavior, and Developmental Disabilities
Achenbach System of Empirically Based Assessment – Preschool Module (ASEBA) Child Behavior Checklist (CBCL/1½ –5) Caregiver-Teacher Report Form (C-TRF)	Achenbach and Rescorla (2000)	1 year 6 months–5 years	Competencies, Strengths, Adaptive Functioning, Behavioral, Emotional and Social Problems
Adaptive Behavior Assessment System – Third Edition (ABAS-3)	Harrison and Oakland (2015)	Birth–89 years 11 months	Adaptive Skills
Adaptive Behavior Diagnostic Scale (ABDS)	Pearson et al. (2016)	2 years–21 years	Conceptual, Social, and Practical
ADHD Symptom Checklist-4 (ADHD-SC4)	Gadow and Sprafkin (2008)	3 years–18 years	Peer Conflict, Stimulant Side Effects, ADHD (Inattentive Type, Hyperactive-Impulsive Type, and Combined Type), ODD

Ages and Stages Questionnaires – Third Edition (ASQ-3)	Squires and Bricker (2009)	1 month–66 months	Communication, Motor (Gross & Fine), Problem Solving, and Personal-Social Skills.
Ages and Stages Questionnaires Social-Emotional – Second Edition (ASQ:SE-2)	Squires et al. (2015)	1 month–72 months	Autonomy, Compliance, Adaptive Functioning, Self-Regulation, Affect, Interaction, and Social-Communication.
Arizona Articulation Proficiency Scale – Fourth Revision (ARIZONA-4)	Fudala and Stegall (2017)	1 year 6 months–18 years	Articulation Proficiency
Asperger Syndrome Diagnostic Scale (ASDS)	Myles et al. (2001)	5 years–18 years	ASD Symptoms
Assessing Linguistic Behavior (ALB)	Olswang et al. (1987)	0–24 months	Play, Communicative Intention, Cognitive Antecedents, Language Production, and Comprehension
Assessment for Persons Profoundly or Severely Impaired – Second Edition (APPSI-2)	Bradley-Johnson et al. (2019)	0–24 months	Alertness, Preferences, Problem-Solving Prerequisites, Communication, and Social–Emotional
Assessment of Children's Language Comprehension, 1983 Revision (ACLC)	Foster et al. (1983)	3 years 0 months–6 years 5 months	Language

(Continued)

Test Name	Author(s) (Year of Publication)	Age Range	Developmental Domains or Areas Assessed
Assessment, Evaluation, and Programming System for Infants and Children, Third Edition (AEPS-3)	Bricker et al. (2022)	Birth and 6 years	Motor (Fine & Gross), Adaptive, Cognitive Social-Emotional, Social-Communication, Literacy, and Math
Attention Deficit Disorders Evaluation Scale – Fifth Edition (ADDED-3)	McCarney and House (2019)	5 years–17 years	ADHD (Inattentive Type, Hyperactive-Impulsive Type, and Combined Type)
Attention-Deficit/Hyperactivity Disorder Test – Second Edition (ADHDT-2)	Gilliam (2015)	5 years–17 years	ADHD and Severity
Auditory Skills Assessment (ASA)	Geffner and Goldman (2010)	3 years 6 months–6 years 11 months	Speech Discrimination, Phonological Awareness, and Nonspeech Processing
Autism Diagnostic Interview – Revised (ADI-R)	Rutter et al. (2003)	3 years–43 years	Communication, Social Development and Play, Repetitive and Restrictive Behaviors, and General Behavior
Autism Diagnostic Observation Scale, Second Edition (ADOS-2)	Lord et al. (2012)	2 years–13 years 11 months	Communication and Social Interaction
Autism Screening Instrument for Educational Planning – Third Edition (ASIEP-3)	Krug et al. (2008)	18 months–adult	Sensory, Relating, Body and Object Use, Language, Social, and Self-Help

Autism Spectrum Rating Scales (ASRS)	Goldstein and Naglieri (2009)	2 years–18 years	Autism Spectrum
Bankson-Bernthal Test of Phonology – Second Edition (BBTOP – 2)	Bankson and Bernthal (2020)	3 years–9 years 11 months	Articulation and Phonological Processing
Bankson Expressive Language Test – Third Edition (BELT-3)	Bankson et al. (2018)	3 years–6 years 11 months	Lexical Semantics, Morphology, and Syntax
Battelle Developmental Inventory, Third Edition (BDI-3)	Newborg (2020)	Birth–7 years 11 months	Cognitive, Adaptive, Communication, Social-Emotional, and Motor
Bayley Infant Neurodevelopmental Screener (BINS)	Aylward (1995)	3 months–24 months	Neurological, Receptive, and Expressive Functions, Processing, and Mental Activity
Bayley Scales of Infant Development – Fourth Edition (Bayley-4)	Bayley and Aylward (2019)	1 month–42 months	Cognitive, Language (Receptive & Expressive), Motor (Gross & Fine), Social-Emotional, Adaptive Behavior, Daily Living Skills, and Socialization
Behavior Assessment System for Children, Third Edition (BASC-3)	Reynolds and Kamphaus (2015b)	2 years–25 years	Social-Emotional, Internal Competencies (Behavior or Emotional Status)
BASC-3 Behavioral and Emotional Screening System (BASC-3 BESS)	Reynolds and Kamphaus (2015a)	3 years–18 years 11 months	Behavioral and Emotional Strengths and Weaknesses

(*Continued*)

Test Name	Author(s) (Year of Publication)	Age Range	Developmental Domains or Areas Assessed
Beery-Buktenica Developmental Test of Visual-Motor Integration, Sixth Edition (Beery VMI)	Beery et al. (2010)	2 years–100 years	Visual-Motor Integration, Visual Perception, and Motor Coordination
Behavioral and Emotional Rating Scale, Second Edition (BERS-2)	Epstein (2004)	5 years–18 years, 11 months	Personal Strengths and Competencies
Behavioral Assessment of Baby's Emotional and Social Style (BABES)	Finello and Poulsen (2018)	Birth–3 years	Social-Emotional
Behavior Rating Inventory of Executive Function, Second Edition (BRIEF-2)	Gioia et al. (2015)	5 years–18 years	Executive Function
Birth to Three Assessment and Intervention System – Second Edition (BTAIS-2)	Ammer and Bangs (2000)	Birth–3 years	Language Comprehension, Language Expression, Nonverbal Thinking, Social/Personal Development, and Motor Development.
Boehm Test of Basic Concepts – Third Edition (Boehm-3)	Boehm (2001)	Grades K–2	Basic Concepts Important for Language and Cognitive Development
Boehm Test of Basic Concepts – 3 Preschool	Boehm (2001)	3 years–5 years 11 months	Basic Relation Concepts in Quality, Spatial, Temporal, and Quantity
Bracken Basic Concept Scale – Fourth Edition (BBCS – 4)	Bracken (2022a)	3 years–7 years 11 months	Receptive Knowledge of Basic Concepts

Bracken School Readiness Assessment, Fourth Edition (BSRA-4)	Bracken (2022b)	3 years–7 years 11 months	School Readiness, Colors, Numbers/Counting, Sizes, Comparisons, and Shapes
Brazelton Neonatal Behavioral Assessment Scale, Fourth Edition	Brazelton and Nugent (2011)	3 days–2 months	Habituation, Orientation, Motor Performance, Range of State, State Regulation, Autonomic Regulation, and Abnormal Reflexes.
Brigance Early Childhood Screens III	Brigance and French (2013)	Birth–7 years 6 months	Physical Development, Language, Academic/Cognitive, Self-Help, and Social-Emotional Skills
Brief Infant/Toddler Social Emotional Assessment (BITSEA)	Briggs-Gowan and Carter (2006)	12 months–36 months	Identify Social-Emotional/Behavioral Problems and Delays in Competence
Brown Attention-Deficit Disorder Scales for Children and Adolescents (Brown ADD Scales for Children)	Brown (2001)	3 years–18 years	Executive Cognitive Functioning
Callier-Azusa Scale	Stillman (1984)	Birth–8 years	Motor, Perceptual, Cognitive, Social, Communication and Language Development, and Daily Living Skills

(Continued)

Test Name	Author(s) (Year of Publication)	Age Range	Developmental Domains or Areas Assessed
Carey Temperament Scales (CTS)	Carey and McDevitt (1995)	1 month–12 years 11 months	Temperament (Activity, Biological Regularity, Adaptability, Approach, Intensity, Mood, Persistence, Distractibility, Threshold)
Carolina Record of Individual Behavior (CRIB)	Simeonsson et al. (1982)	Birth–6 years	Sensorimotor
Carrow Elicited Language Inventory (CELI)	Carrow-Woolfolk (1974)	3 years–7 years	Language Skills and Grammar
Cattell Infant Intelligence Scale	Cattell (1940)	3 months–30 months	Willingness, Self-Confidence, Social-Confidence, Attention
Checklist for Autism in Toddlers-23 (CHAT-23)	Wong et al. (2004)	Mental ages 18–24 months	Gaze monitoring, Pretend Play, Protodeclarative Pointing
Child and Adolescent Memory Profile (ChAMP)	Sherman and Brooks (2015)	5 years–21 years	Visual and Verbal Memory
Child Development Inventories (CDI)	Ireton (1992)	1 year 3 months–6 years 3 months	Social, Self-Help, Motor (Gross & Fine), Language, Letters, and Numbers
Childhood Autism Rating Scale, Second Edition – Standard Version (CARS2-ST)	Schopler et al. (2010)	2 years and older	Adaptive Skills, Social and Emotional Functioning

Clinical Assessment of Articulation and Phonology – Second Edition (CAAP-2)	Secord and Donohue (2013)	3 years–11 years 11 months	Articulation and Phonology
Clinical Assessment of Behavior (CAB)	Bracken and Keith (2004)	2 years–18 years	Psychosocial Strengths and Weaknesses, and Adjustment
Clinical Assessment of Language Comprehension	Miller and Paul (1995)	8 months–10 years	Language Comprehension
Clinical Evaluation of Language Fundamentals Preschool, Third Edition (CELF Preschool -3)	Wiig et al. (2020)	3 years–6 years 11 months	Receptive Language and Expressive Language
Cognitive Assessment of Young Children (CAYC)	Langley et al. (2010)	2 months–5 years 11 months	Fine Motor Coordination and Planning, Communication and Play, Memory, Reasoning, Perceptual Development, Processing, Classification and Organization, Concept Development, and Practical Knowledge
Cognitive Abilities Scale: Second Edition (CAS-2)	Bradley-Johnson and Johnson (2001)	3 months–47 months	Adaptive Behavior
Communication and Symbolic Behavior Scales Developmental Profile: First Normed Edition (CSBS-DP)	Wetherby and Prizant (2002)	6 months–24 months	Emotion and Eye Gaze, Communications, Gestures, Language
Comprehensive Assessment of Spoken Language, Second Edition	Carrow-Woolfolk (2017)	3 years–21 years	Oral Language Processing

(Continued)

Test Name	Author(s) (Year of Publication)	Age Range	Developmental Domains or Areas Assessed
Comprehensive Receptive and Expressive Vocabulary Test – Third Edition (CREVT – 3)	Wallace and Hammill (2013)	4 years–18 years	Receptive and Expressive Vocabulary
Comprehensive Test of Phonological Processing – Second Edition (CTOPP-2)	Wagner et al. (2013)	4 years–24 years, 11 months	Phonological Awareness, Phonological Memory, and Rapid Naming
Coping Inventory: A Measure of Adaptive Behavior	Zeitlin (1985)	3–adult	Coping and Adaptive Behavior
The Capute Scales; Cognitive Adaptive Test/ Clinical Linguistic and Auditory Milestone Scales (CAT/CLAMS)	Accardo and Capute (2005)	1 month–36 months	Language, Problem Solving, and Visual-Motor Skills.
Denver Developmental Screening Test – Second Edition (Denver II)	Frankenburg et al. (1992)	Birth–6 years	Gross Motor, Language, Fine Motor-Adaptive, Personal-Social, and Behavior.
Detroit Tests of Learning Aptitude-Primary, Third Edition (DTLA-P:3)	Hammill and Bryant (2005)	3 months–9 years 11 months	Cognitive, Language, Attention, and Motor Abilities
Development Test of Visual Perception – Third Edition (DTVP-3)	Hammill et al. (2013)	4 years–12 years, 11 months	Visual Perception and Visual-Motor
Developmental Activities Screening Inventory – Second Edition (DASI-II)	Fewell and Langley (1984)	Birth–5 years	Perceptual, Motor, and Cognitive Skills

Developmental Assessment for Individuals with Severe Disabilities – Third Edition (DASH-3)	Dykes and Mruzek (2012)	Functioning at Level of Birth to 7 years	Sensory-Motor, Language, Social-Emotional, Activities of Daily Living, and Academics
Developmental Assessment of Young Children – Second Edition (DAYC-2)	Voress et al. (2012)	Birth–5 years	Cognitive, Communication, Social-Emotional, Physical Development, and Adaptive Behavior
Developmental Behavior Checklist 2 (DBC2)	Gray et al. (2018)	4 years–18 years	Development
Developmental Indicators for the Assessment of Learning – Fourth Edition (DIAL-4)	Mardell and Goldenberg (2011)	2 years 6 months–5 years 11 months	Visual, Motor, Quantitative Concepts, Language, Self-Help, Personal Information, and Social-Emotional Skills
Developmental Programming for Infants and Young Children – Revised Edition	Schafer and Moersch (1981)	Birth–60 months	Fine Motor, Cognition, Language, Social-Emotional, Self-Care, and Gross Motor
Developmental Profile 4 (DP-4)	Alpern (2020)	Birth–21 years 11 months	Physical, Adaptive Behavior, Social-Emotional, Cognitive, and Communication
Devereux Early Childhood Assessment-Clinical Form (DECA-C)	LeBuffe and Naglieri (2002)	2 years–5 years 11 months	Initiative, Self-Control, Withdrawal/Depression, Emotional Control, Attention, Aggression and Attachment

(Continued)

Test Name	Author(s) (Year of Publication)	Age Range	Developmental Domains or Areas Assessed
Devereux Early Childhood Assessment for Preschoolers, Second Edition (DECA-P2)	LeBuffe and Naglieri (2012)	3 years–6 years	Initiative, Self-Regulation, and Attachment
Devereux Early Childhood Assessment for Infants and Toddlers (DECA-I/T)	MacKrain and LeBuffe (2007)	1 month–36 months	Initiative, Attachment/ Relationships, and Self-Regulation
Diagnostic Evaluation of Articulation and Phonology (DEAP)	Dodd et al. (2006)	3 years–8 years 11 months	Language
Diagnostic Evaluation of Language Variation – Normed Referenced	Seymour et al. (2018)	4 years–9 years 11 months	Syntax, Pragmatics, Semantics, and Phonology
Differential Ability Scales – Second Edition (DAS-II)	Elliott (2007)	2 years 6 months–17 years 11 months	Cognitive Abilities
Dynamic Indicators of Basic Early Literacy Education – Eighth Edition (DIBELS)	University of Oregon (2023)	Grades K–8	Early Literacy Skills
Dynamic Assessment and Intervention: Improving Children's Narrative Abilities	Miller et al. (2001)	Preschool–elementary school	Storytelling Ability
Early Childhood Inventory-5 (ECI-5)	Gadow and Sprafkin (2013)	3 years–5 years	Symptoms of Childhood Disorders
Early Coping Inventory	Zeitlin et al. (1988)	Mental age 4 months–36 months	Sensorimotor Organization, Reactive Behaviors, Self-Initiated Behaviors

Early Functional Communication Profile (EFCP)	Jensen (2012)	2 years–10 years	Joint Attention, Social Interaction, Communicative Intent, Social Interaction, and Joint Attention
Early Language Milestone Scale – Second Edition (ELM Scale – 2)	Coplan (1993)	0 months–36 months	Auditory Expressive, Auditory Receptive, and Visual Skills
Early Screening Inventory, Third Edition (ESI-3)	Meisels et al. (2019)	3 years–5 years 11 months	Visual Motor/Adaptive, Language and Cognition, and Gross Motor Skills.
Early Screening Project (ESP)	Walker et al. (1995)	3 years–6 years	Aggressive Behavior, Social Interaction, Adaptive/ Maladaptive Behavior
Early Screening Profiles (ESP)	Harrison et al. (1990)	2 years–6 years 11 months	Cognitive/Language, Motor, Self-Help/Social, Articulation, and Behavior
Emotional Disturbance Decision Tree (EDDT)	Euler (2007)	5 years–18 years	Emotional Disturbance
Expressive One-Word Picture Vocabulary Test, Fourth Edition (EOWPVT-4)	Martin and Brownell (2011a)	2 years–70+ years	Expressive Vocabulary
Expressive Vocabulary Test – Third Edition (EVT-3)	Williams (2019)	2 years 6 months– 90+ years	Expressive Vocabulary

(Continued)

Test Name	Author(s) (Year of Publication)	Age Range	Developmental Domains or Areas Assessed
Evaluating Acquired Skills in Communication – Third Edition (EASIC-3)	Marcott (2009)	3 months–6 years	Prelinguistic Skills, Semantics, Syntax, Morphology, and Pragmatics
Eyberg Child Behavior Inventory (ECBI) and the Sutter-Eyberg Student Behavior Inventory – Revised (SESBI- R)	Eyberg and Pincus (1999)	2 years–16 years	Conduct Behavior Problems
FirstSTEP: Screening Test for Evaluating Preschoolers	Miller (1993)	2 years 9 months–6 years 2 months	Cognition, Communication, Motor, Social-Emotional, and Adaptive Behavior
Fluharty Preschool Speech and Language Screening Test – Second Edition (FLUHARTY-2)	Fluharty (2000)	3 years–6 years 11 months	Articulation and Language (Receptive, Expressive, and Composite)
Functional Communication Profile Revised (FCP-R)	Kleiman (2003)	3 years–adult	Communication Skills
Functional Emotional Assessment Scale (FEAS)	Greenspan et al. (2001)	7 months–48 months	Emotional Functioning
Gesell Developmental Observation – Revised	Gesell Institute of Child Development (2012)	1 week–36 months	Adaptive, Motor (Gross & Fine), Language, and Personal-Social
Gesell School Readiness Test (GSRT)	Ilg et al. (1978)	2 years 6 months–6 years 11 months	Adaptive and Language Development

Gilliam Asperger's Disorder Scale (GADS)	Gilliam (2001)	3 years–22 years	Social Interaction, Restricted Patterns, Cognitive Patterns, and Pragmatic Skills.
Gilliam Autism Rating Scale – Third Edition (GARS-3)	Gilliam (2014)	3 years–22 years	Stereotyped Behaviors, Communication, Emotional Responses, and Social Interaction
Goldman-Fristoe Test of Articulation, Third Edition (GFTA-3)	Goldman and Fristoe (2015)	2 years–21 years 11 months	Articulation
Greenspan Social-Emotional Growth Chart	Greenspan (2004)	Birth–3 years 6 months	Social-Emotional
Griffiths Scales of Child Development, Third Edition (Griffiths III)	Stroud et al. (2016)	Birth–6 years	Foundations of Learning, Language, Hand-eye Coordination, Social-Emotional, and Gross Motor
Hawaii Early Learning Profiles: 3–6 Years, Second Edition (HELP: 3–6)	VORT Corporation (2010)	3 years–6 years	Regulatory/Sensory Organization, Cognitive, Language, Gross/Fine Motor, Social-Emotional, Self-Help
Revised Hiskey-Nebraska Test of Learning Aptitude (H-NTLA)	Hiskey (1966)	3 years–17 years	Visual Attention, Memory, Classification, Spatial Reasoning, Eye-Hand Coordination
Hodson Assessment of Phonological Patterns – Third Edition (HAPP-3)	Hodson (2004)	3 years–8 years	Phonological Patterns

(*Continued*)

Test Name	Author(s) (Year of Publication)	Age Range	Developmental Domains or Areas Assessed
Howes Peer Play Scale (Revised)	Howes and Matheson (1992)	Toddler–59 months	Parallel Play, Parallel Aware Play, Simple Social Play, Complementary and Reciprocal Play, and Complex Social Pretend Play
Infant Development Inventory (IDI)	Ireton (1994)	Birth–18 months	Social, Self-Help, Gross-Motor, Fine Motor, and Language
Infant-Toddler and Family Instrument (IFTI)	Provence and Apfel (2001)	6 months–3 years	Motor (Gross & Fine) Social-Emotional, Language, Coping, and Self-Help
Infant-Toddler Developmental Assessment – Second Edition (IDA-2)	Provence et al. (2016)	Birth–36 months	Motor (Gross & Fine), Relationship to Inanimate Objects/Cognition, Language/Communication, Self-Help/Adaptive, Relationship to Persons, Emotions and Feeling States, and Coping Behavior
Infant-Toddler and Brief Infant-Toddler Social and Emotional Assessment (BITSEA; ITSEA)	Briggs-Gowan and Carter (2002)	12 months–36 months	Social-Emotional
Infant/Toddler Sensory Profile	Dunn (2002)	Birth–36 months	Sensory processing ability

Instrument	Author (year)	Age range	Areas assessed
Infant-Toddler Symptom Checklist: A Screening Tool for Parents	DeGangi et al. (1995)	7 months–30 months	Self-Regulation, Attention, Sleep, Eating/Feeding, Dressing, Bathing and Touch, Movement, Listening and Language, Looking and Sight, and Attachment/Emotional Functioning
Iowa Tests of Basic Skills (ITBS)	Hoover et al. (2003)	Grades K–9	Content Areas of School Curricula
Kaufman Assessment Battery for Children: Second Edition Normative Update (KABC-II NU)	Kaufman and Kaufman (2018)	3 years–18 years	Cognitive Abilities
Kaufman Brief Intelligence Test, Second Edition, Revised (KBIT-2 Revised)	Kaufman and Kaufman (2022)	4 years–90 years	Verbal and Nonverbal Skills
Kaufman Speech Praxis Test for Children (KSPT)	Kaufman (2016)	2 years–5 years 11 months	Speech and Language Pathology
Kaufman Survey of Early Academic and Language Skills (K-SEALS)	Kaufman and Kaufman (1993)	3 years–6 years 11 months	School Readiness, Language Skills, Pre-Academic Skills, and Articulation
Kent Inventory of Developmental Skills (KIDS)	Reuter et al. (2000)	Birth–15 months or up to age 6 when severe developmental disabilities are present	Cognitive, Motor, Communication, Self-Help, Social Skills
Khan-Lewis Phonological Analysis – Third Edition (KLPA-3)	Khan and Lewis (2015)	2 years–21 years 11 months	Phonological Processes

(Continued)

Test Name	Author(s) (Year of Publication)	Age Range	Developmental Domains or Areas Assessed
Koppitz Developmental Scoring System for the Bender Gestalt Test, Second Edition (Koppitz-2)	Reynolds (2007)	5 years–85 years	Visual-Motor Integration Skills
Learning Accomplishment Profile Diagnostic Edition (LAP-D) Third Edition	Hardin et al. (2005)	Birth–6 years	Fine Motor Manipulation, Fine Motor Writing, Cognitive Matching, Cognitive Counting, Language Naming, Language comprehension, Gross Motor Body Movement, and Gross Motor Object Movement
Leiter International Performance Scale, Third Edition (Leiter–3)	Roid et al. (2013)	3 years–75 years+	Reasoning, Visualization, Memory, and Attention.
Lindamood Auditory Conceptualization Test – Third Edition (LAC-3)	Lindamood and Lindamood (2004)	5 years–18 years 11 months	Speech and Language Development
MacArthur-Bates Communicative Development Inventories (MB-CDIs)	Fenson et al. (2007)	1 year–3 years	Comprehension and Talking
MacArthur Story Stem Battery (MSSB)	Bretherton (1990)	3 years–7 years	Attachment, Response to Authority, Response to Family Conflict, Response to Getting Caught Doing a Transgression, and Separation Anxiety
McCarthy Scales of Children's Abilities (MSCA)	McCarthy (1972)	2 years 6 months–8 years 6 months	Cognitive and Motor Behaviors

Instrument	Source	Age Range	Domains Assessed
Meadow/Kendall Social-Emotional Assessment Inventories for Deaf and Hearing-Impaired Students Preschool Form (SEAI)	Meadow et al. (1983)	3–6 years 11 months	Communication
Mental Health Screening Tool (MHST 0–5)	The California Institute for Mental Health (2000)	Birth–5 years	Social-Emotional
Merill-Palmer – R Scales of Development (M-P-R)	Roid and Sampers (2004)	Birth–6 years 5 months	Cognitive, Language, Motor (Fine & Gross), Social-Emotional, and Self-Help
Metropolitan Readiness Test, Sixth Edition (MRT6)	Nurss and McGauvran (1995)	Pre-K–Grade 1	Basic and Advanced Language and Mathematics Skills
Milani-Comparetti Motor Development Screening Test	Stuberg et al. (1992)	1 month–16 months	Motor Function
Miller Assessment for Preschoolers (MAP)	Miller (1982)	2 years 9 months–5 years 8 months	Motor, Language, and Cognition
Miller Function and Participation Scales (M-FUN)	Miller (2006)	2 years–7 years 11 months	Motor
Modified Checklist for Autism in Toddlers, Revised, with Follow-Up (M-CHAT-R/F)	Robins et al. (2009)	16 months–30 months	Protodeclarative Pointing, Gaze Monitoring, and Pretend Play
Monteiro Interview Guidelines for Diagnosing the Autism Spectrum, Second Edition (MIGDAS-2)	Monteiro and Stegall (2018)	3 years–99 years	Individual's Interaction with Environment

(Continued)

Test Name	Author(s) (Year of Publication)	Age Range	Developmental Domains or Areas Assessed
Motor-Free Visual Perception Test – 4 (MVPT-4)	Colarusso and Hammill (2015)	4 years–80 years	Visual Perceptual
Movement Assessment Battery for Children – Third Edition (MABC –3)	Henderson and Barnett (2023)	3 years–25 years	Coordination, Fine and Gross Motor
Mullen Scales of Early Learning: AGS Edition	Mullen (1995)	Birth–68 months	Gross Motor (birth to 33 months only), Fine Motor, Visual Reception, Receptive Language, and Expressive Language
NEPSY – Second Edition (NEPSY-II)	Korkman et al. (2007)	3 years–16 years 11 months	Executive Functioning/ Attention, Language, Memory/ Learning, Sensorimotor Functioning, Visuospatial Processing, and Social Perception
Northwestern Syntax Screening Test (NSST)	Lee (1971)	3 years–7 years 11 months	Identify Language Deficiencies
Oral and Written Language Scales – Second Edition (OWLS-II)	Carrow-Woolfolk (2011)	3 years–21 years 11 months	Oral Language, Written Language, Receptive Processing and Expressive Processing
Oral-Motor/Feeding Rating Scale	Jelm (1990)	All ages	Oral-Motor and Feeding (i.e., breastfeeding, bottle feeding, spoon feeding, cup drinking, and chewing)

Parent Interview for Autism – Clinical Version (PIA-CV)	Stone et al. (2003)	Under the age of 3 years	Communication, Language, Social Relating, Affective Responses, Sensory, Motor, Play, and Behavior Skills, and Need for Sameness
Parents' Evaluations of Developmental Status- Revised (PEDS-R)	Glascoe et al. (2023)	Birth–7 years 11 months	Language, Motor, Self-Help, Early Academic Skills, Behavior and Social-Emotional/Mental Health
Peabody Developmental Motor Scales – Third Edition (PDMS-3)	Folio and Fewell (2023)	Birth–5 years	Body Control, Body Transport, Object Control, and Eye-Hand Coordination
Peabody Picture Vocabulary Test – Fifth Edition (PPVT-5)	Dunn (2018)	2 years 6 months–90+ years	Receptive and Expressive Vocabulary Acquisition
Pediatric Evaluation of Disability (PEDI)	Haley et al. (1992)	6 months–7 years	Self-Care, Mobility, and Social Function
Pediatric Evaluation of Disability Inventory Computer Adaptive Test (PEDI-CAT)	Haley et al. (2020)	1 month–20 years 11 months	Daily Activities, Mobility, Social, and Cognition
Penn Interactive Peer Play Scale (PIPPS)	Fantuzzo et al (1995)	Preschool children	Play Interaction, Play Disruption, and Play Disconnection
Personality Inventory for Children – Second Edition (PIC-2)	Lachar and Gruber (2002)	5 years–19 years	Emotional, Behavioral, Social, and Cognitive Adjustment

(Continued)

Test Name	Author(s) (Year of Publication)	Age Range	Developmental Domains or Areas Assessed
Pervasive Developmental Disorders Screening Test, Second Edition (PDDST-II)	Siegel (2004)	12 months–48 months	Behavior Development
Photo Articulation Test – Third Edition (PAT-3)	Lippke et al. (1997)	3–8 years 11 months	Speech Analysis
Preschool and Kindergarten Behavior Scales – Second Edition (PKBS-2)	Merrell (2002)	3 years–6 years	Social Skills and Problem Behavior (Externalizing & Internalizing).
Preschool Behavior Checklist	Richman (1988)	2 years–5 years 11 months	Behavior and Emotional Difficulties
Preschool Behavior Questionnaire (PBQ)	Behar and Stringfield (1974)	3 years–6 years	Emotional Problems
Preschool Child Observation Record – Second Edition (COR)	Barton (2023)	2 years 6 months–6 years	Initiative, Social Relations, Creative Representation, Movement and Music, Language and Literacy, and Mathematics and Science
Preschool Language Assessment Instrument – Second Edition (PLAI-2)	Blank et al. (2003)	3 years–5 years 11 months	Matching, Analysis, Reordering, Reasoning, Receptive Mode, and Expressive Mode

Assessment	Author	Age Range	Skills Assessed
Preschool Language Scale – Fifth Edition (PLS-5)	Zimmerman et al. (2011)	Birth–7 years 11 months	Auditory Comprehension and Expressive Communication
Pre-Literacy Skills Screening (PLSS)	Crumrine and Lonegan (1999)	3 years–5 years 11 months	Letter Knowledge, Phonological Awareness, and Reading Readiness Skills
Primary Test of Nonverbal Intelligence (PTONI)	Ehrler and McGhee (2008)	3 years–9 years 11 months	Cognitive Skills
Psychoeducational Profile: TEACCH Individualized Psychoeducational Assessment for Children with Autism Spectrum Disorders – Third Edition (PEP-3)	Schopler et al. (2005)	2–7 years 6 months, or children functioning within this age range	Education Planning and ASD Diagnosis
Receptive One-Word Picture Vocabulary Test – Fourth Edition (ROWPVT-4)	Martin and Brownell (2011b)	2 years–70+years	Receptive Vocabulary Skills
Receptive Expressive Emergent Language Test – Fourth Edition (REEL-4)	Brown et al. (2020)	Birth–3 years	Receptive and Expressive Language
Receptive, Expressive & Social Communication Assessment – Elementary (RESCA-E)	Hamaguchi and Ross-Swain (2015)	5 years–12 years	Receptive, Expressive, and Social Language Development
New Reynell Developmental Language Scales (NRDLS)	Edwards et al. (2011)	3 years–7 years 6 months	Expressive Language and Verbal Comprehension

(Continued)

Test Name	Author(s) (Year of Publication)	Age Range	Developmental Domains or Areas Assessed
Reynell-Zinkin Scales: Developmental Scales for Young Visually Handicapped	Reynell (1979)	Birth–5 years	Social Adaptation, Sensorimotor, Exploration of Environment, Response to Sound/Verbal Comprehension, Expressive Language and Nonverbal Communication
Reynolds Intellectual Assessment Scales, Second Edition (RIAS-2)	Reynolds and Kamphaus (2015c)	3 years–94 years	Verbal Intelligence, Nonverbal Intelligence, and Memory
Rossetti Infant-Toddler Language Scale	Rossetti (2006)	Birth–3 years	Preverbal and Verbal Communication
Scales of Independent Behavior – Revised (SIB-R)	Bruininks et al. (1996)	3 months–80+ years	Motor, Social/Communication, Personal Independence, and Community
Screening Tool for Autism in Toddlers & Young Children (STAT)	Stone and Ousley (2008)	24 months–36 months	Play, Imitation, Directing Attention, and (not scored) Response to Requests
Sensory Processing Measure –Second Edition, Preschool (SPM-2)	Parham (2021)	2 years–5 years	Social Participation, Vision, Hearing, Touch, Body Awareness, Balance and Motion, Planning and Ideas, and Total Sensory Systems
Sensory Profile 2	Dunn (2014)	Birth–14 years 11 months	Sensory

Measure	Citation	Age Range	Construct
Sequenced Inventory of Communication Development – Revised (SICD-R)	Hedrick et al. (1984)	4 months–4 years	Communication Skills (Receptive and Expressive)
Slosson Intelligence Test – Fourth Edition (SIT-4)	Slosson (2017)	4 years–65 years	Cognitive Ability
Smith-Johnson Nonverbal Performance Scale	Smith and Johnson (1977)	2 years–4 years	Cognitive Skills
Social Communication Questionnaire (SCQ)	Rutte et al. (2003)	4 years–40 years	Social Development and Play, Communication, and Repetitive and Restrictive Behavior Domains on the ADI-R
Social Competence and Behavior Evaluation Preschool Edition (SCBE)	LaFreniere and Dumas (1995)	2 years 6 months–6 years	Social Skills
Social Emotional Assets and Resilience Scales (SEARS)	Merrell (2011)	5 years–18 years	Self-Regulation, Responsibility, Social Competence, and Empathy
Social Responsiveness Scale – Second Edition (SRS-2)	Constantino (2012)	3 years–99 years	Social (Awareness, Cognition, Communication, Motivation), Restricted Interests and Repetitive Behavior
Social Skills Improvement System (SSIS) Rating Scales	Gresham and Elliott (2008)	3 years–18 years	Communication, Engagement, Bullying, and Autism Spectrum

(*Continued*)

Test Name	Author(s) (Year of Publication)	Age Range	Developmental Domains or Areas Assessed
Social Skills Rating System (SSRS)	Gresham and Elliott (1990)	3 years–18 years	Social Skills, Problem Behavior (Externalizing & Internalizing), Hyperactivity, and Academic Competence
Stanford-Binet Intelligence Scales –Fifth Edition (SB-5)	Roid (2003)	2 years–85+ years	Fluid Reasoning, Knowledge, Quantitative Reasoning, Visual-Spatial Processing, and Working Memory
Strengths and Difficulties Questionnaire (SDQ)	Goodman (1997)	2 years–17 years	Emotional Symptoms, Conduct Problems, Hyperactivity/Inattention, Peer Relationship Problems, Prosocial Behavior
Structured Photographic Expressive Language Test – Preschool Second Edition (SPELT-P 2)	Dawson et al. (2005)	3 years–5 years 11 months	Diagnose Language Impairment
Stuttering Severity Instrument – Fourth Edition (SSI-4)	Riley (2009)	2 years–10 years and older	Speech Development
Symbolic Play Scale Checklist	Westby (2000)	Birth–5 years (and older children with learning problems)	Decontextualization, Thematic Content, Organization, Self-Other Relations, and Language
Symbolic Play Test - Second Edition	Lowe and Costello (1988)	1 year–3 years	Cognitive and Expressive Language

Assessment	Author(s)	Age Range	Areas Assessed
A Language Processing Skills Assessment (TAPS-4)	Martin et al. (2018)	5 years–21 years	Phonological Processing, Auditory Memory, and Listening Comprehension
Temperament and Atypical Behavior Scale (TABS)	Bagnato et al. (1999)	11 months–71 months	Atypical Self-Regulatory Behavior
Test for Auditory Comprehension of Language – Fourth Edition (TACL-4)	Carrow-Woolfolk (2014)	3 years–12 years 11 months	Vocabulary, Grammatical Morphemes, Phrases, and Sentences
Test Observation Form (TOF)	McConaughy and Achenbach (2004)	2 years–18 years	Behavior, Affect, and Test-Taking Style During Testing Sessions
Test of Early Communication and Emerging Language (TECEL)	Huer and Miller (2011)	2 weeks–24 months or older if the child has moderate to severe language delays	Receptive and Expressive Language
Test of Early Language Development - Fourth Edition (TELD-4)	Hresko et al. (2018)	3 years–7 years, 11 months	Language
Test of Early Mathematics Ability – Third Edition (TEMA-3)	Ginsburg and Baroody (2003)	3 years–8 years 11 months	Numbering Skills, Number-Comparison Facility, Numeral Literacy, Mastery of Number Facts, Calculation Skills, and Understanding of Concepts
Test of Early Reading Ability – Deaf or Hard of Hearing (TERA-D/HH)	Reid et al. (1991)	3 years–13 years 11 months	Early Reading

(Continued)

Test Name	Author(s) (Year of Publication)	Age Range	Developmental Domains or Areas Assessed
Test of Early Reading Ability – Fourth Edition (TERA-4)	Reid et al. (2018)	4 years–8 years 11 months	Alphabet, Conventions, and Meaning
Test of Gross Motor Development – Third Edition (TGMD-3)	Ulrich (2019)	3 years–10 years 11 months	Gross Motor Skill Development
Test of Information Processing Skills (TIPS)	Webster (2009)	5 years–90 years	Visual and Auditory Processing
Test of Irregular Word Reading Efficiency (TIWRE)	Reynolds and Kamphaus (2007)	3 years–94 years	Reading Comprehension
Tests of Phonological Awareness – Second Edition: PLUS (TOPA-2+)	Torgesen and Bryant (2004)	5 years–8 years	Phonological Awareness and Relationship Between Letter and Phonemes in English
Test of Visual-Motor Skills – Third Edition (TVMS-3)	Martin (2010)	3 years–90+ years	Visual Perception, Motor Planning, and/or Execution
Test of Visual Perceptual Skills – 4 (TVPS-4)	Martin (2017)	5 years–21 years	Visual Analysis and Visual Processing Skills
The Ounce Scale	Meisels et al. (2003)	Birth–3 years 6 months	Personal Connections, Feelings About Self, Relationships with Other Children, Understanding and Communication, Exploration and Problem Solving, Movement and Coordination

The Temperament Assessment Battery for Children (TABC)	Martin (1988)	3 years–7 years	Activity, Adaptability, Approach/Withdrawal, Emotional Intensity, Distractibility, and Persistence
Token Test for Children – Second Edition (TTFC-2)	McGhee et al. (2007)	3 years–12 years 11 months	Receptive Language
Transdisciplinary Play-Based Assessment, Second Edition (TPBA2)	Linder (2008)	Birth–6 years	Cognitive Abilities, Social-Emotional Functioning, Communication and Language Skills, and Sensory-Motor Development
Universal Nonverbal Intelligence Test, Second Edition (UNIT-2)	Bracken and McCallum (2016)	5 years–21 years 11 months	General Intelligence
Uzgiris-Hunt Ordinal Scales of Psychological Developmental Scale	Uzgiris and Hunt (1975)	2 weeks–2 years	Object Permanence, Use of Objects as Means, Learning and Foresight, Development of Schemata, Development of an Understanding of Causality, Conception of Objects in Space, Vocal Imitation, and Gestural Imitation
Verbal Behavior Milestones Assessment and Placement Program (VB-MAPP) Second Edition	Sundberg (2016)	Birth–48 months	Language and Social Skills

(*Continued*)

Test Name	Author(s) (Year of Publication)	Age Range	Developmental Domains or Areas Assessed
Vineland Adaptive Behavior Scales, Third Edition (Vineland-3)	Sparrow et al. (2016)	Birth–90 years	Communication, Daily Living Skills, Socialization, and Motor Skills
Vineland Social – Emotional Early Childhood Scales (SEEC)	Sparrow et al. (1998)	Birth–5 years 11 months	Social and Emotional Functioning
Wechsler Preschool and Primary Scale of Intelligence, Fourth Edition (WPPSI-IV)	Wechsler (2012)	2 years 6 months–7 years 7 months	Cognitive Ability
Wide Range Assessment of Visual Motor Abilities (WRAVMA)	Adams and Sheslow (1995)	3 years–17 years	Visual-Spatial, Visual-Motor, and Fine Motor
Woodcock-Johnson – Fourth Edition (WJ)	Woodcock et al. (2014)	2 years–90 years	Academic Achievement, Oral Language, Scholastic Aptitude, and Overall Cognitive Skills.
Woodcock-Johnson – Fourth Edition Tests of Early Cognitive & Academic Development (WJ-IV ECAD)	Schrank et al. (2015)	2 years 6 months–7 years 11 months	General Intellectual Ability, Early Academic Skills, and Oral Expression
Work Sampling System – Fifth Edition, for Head Start	Dichtelmiller et al. (2014)	Grades Preschool–3	Art and Fine Motor, Movement and Gross Motor, Concept and Number, Language and Literacy, and Personal and Social Development

Note: Although many tests have gone through several revisions, only current editions of each test are referenced here due to space limitations.

REFERENCES

Accardo, P. J., & Capute, A. J. (2005). *The Capute scales: Cognitive adaptive test/clinical linguistic and auditory milestone scale (CAT/CLAMS)*. Paul H. Brookes Publishing.

Achenbach, T. M., & Rescorla, L. A. (2000). *Manual for the ASEBA preschool forms & profiles: An integrated system of multi-informant assessment; Child behavior checklist for ages 1 1/2–5; Language development survey; Caregiver-Teacher report form*. University of Vermont.

Adams, W., & Sheslow, D. (1995). *Wide range assessment of visual motor abilities (WRAVMA) manual*. Psychological Assessment Resources.

Alpern, G. D. (2020). *Developmental profile 4*. WPS.

Ammer, J. J., & Bangs, T. (2000). *Birth to three assessment and intervention system-Second edition*. PRO-ED.

Aylward, G. P. (1995). *Bayley infant neurodevelopmental screener*. Psychological Corporation.

Bagnato, S. J., Neisworth, J. T., Salvia, J., & Hunt, F. M. (1999). *Temperament and atypical behavior scale (TABS) assessment tool*. Brookes Publishing.

Bankson, N. W., & Bernthal, J. E. (2020). *Bankson-Bernthal test of phonology*. PRO-ED.

Bankson, N. W., Mentis, M., & Jagielko, J. R. (2018). *BELT-3: Bankson Expressive Language Test*. PRO-ED.

Barton, H. (2023). *Preschool child observation record—second edition (COR)*. Highscope Press.

Bayley, N., & Aylward, G. P. (2019). *Bayley-4: Scales of infant and toddler development, technical manual* (4th ed.). Pearson.

Beery, K. E., Buktenica, N. A., & Beery, N. A. (2010). *The Beery–Buktenica developmental test of visual–motor integration: Administration, scoring, and teaching manual* (6th ed.). Pearson.

Behar, L., & Stringfield, S. (1974). A behavior rating scale for the preschool child. *Developmental Psychology, 10*(5), 601–610.

Blank, M., Rose, S. A., & Berlin, L. J. (2003). *Preschool language assessment instrument* (2nd ed.). PRO-ED.

Boehm, A. E. (2001). *Boehm test of basic concepts preschool* (3rd ed.). Pearson Education.

Bracken, B. A., & Keith, L. K. (2004). *Professional manual for the clinical assessment of behavior*. Psychological Assessment Resources.

Bracken, B. A., & McCallum, R. S. (2016). *Universal nonverbal intelligence test* (2nd ed.). Riverside.

Bracken, B. A. (2022a). *Bracken basic concept scale* (4th ed.). Pearson Education.

Bracken, B. A. (2022b). *Bracken school readiness assessment, Fourth edition (BSRA-4)*. Pearson Education.

Bradley-Johnson, S., Johnson, C. M., Connard, P., Arick, J. R., & Krug, D. A. (2019). *Assessment for persons with profound or severe impairments* (2nd ed.). PRO-ED.

Bradley-Johnson, S., & Johnson, C. M. (2001). *Cognitive abilities scale* (2nd ed.). PRO-ED.

Brazelton, T. B., & Nugent, J. K. (2011). *Neonatal behavioral assessment scale* (4th ed.). Mac Keith Press.

Bretherton, I. (1990). *MacArthur story-stem battery (MSSB) [Database record]*. APA PsycTests. https://doi.org/10.1037/t05279-000

Bricker, D., Dionne, C., Grisham, J., Johnson, J. J., Macy, M., Slentz, K. L., & Waddell, M. (2022). *Assessment, evaluation, and programming system for infants and young children (AEPS-3)* (3rd ed.). Paul H. Brookes Publishing.

Brigance, A. H., & French, B. (2013). *Brigance early childhood screens III*. Curriculum Associates, LLC.

Briggs-Gowan, M. J., & Carter, A. S. (2002). *Brief infant-toddler social and emotional assessment (BITSEA) manual (Version 2.0)*. Yale University.

Briggs-Gowan, M. J., & Carter, A. S. (2006). *Brief infant-toddler social-emotional assessment (BITSEA)*. APA PsycTests.

Brown, E. T. (2001). *Brown attention-deficit disorder scales*. Pearson Education.

Brown, V. L., Bzoch, K., & League, R. (2020). *Receptive expressive emergent language scales (REEL-4)* (4th ed.). PRO-ED.

Bruininks, R., Woodcock, R. W., Weatherman, R. F., & Hill, B. K. (1996). *Scales of independent behavior-revised (SIB-R)*. Riverside.

California Institute for Mental Health. (2000). Mental health screening tool (MHST): 0 to 5. Retrieved from http://www.earlychildhoodmentalhealth-sandiego.com/wp-content/uploads/2015/09/C-6_-Cosico-Berge_-MHST-0-5_Screening-Tool.pdf (accessed September 23, 2024).

Carey, W. B., & McDevitt, S. C. (1995). *The Carey temperament scales*. Behavioral-Developmental Initiatives.

Carrow-Woolfolk, E. (1974). *Carrow elicited language inventory*. DLM Teaching Resources.

Carrow-Woolfolk, E. (2011). *Oral and written language scales* (2nd ed.). Pearson PsychCorp.

Carrow-Woolfolk, E. (2014). *Test for auditory comprehension of language* (4th ed.). PRO-ED.

Carrow-Woolfolk, E. (2017). *CASL-2: Comprehensive assessment of spoken language* (2nd ed.). Western Psychological Services.

Cattell, P. (1940). *The measurement of intelligence of infants and young children*. Psychological Corporation.

Colarusso, R., & Hammill, D. (2015). *Motor-free visual perception test* (4th ed.). Academic Therapy Publications.

Constantino, J. N. (2012). *The social responsiveness scale* (2nd ed.). Western Psychological Services.

Coplan, J. (1993). *Early language milestone scale: Examiner's manual*. PRO-ED.

Crumrine, L., & Lonegan, H. (1999). *Pre-literacy skills screening*. PRO-ED.

Dawson, J. I., Stout, C. E., Eyer, J. A., Tattersall, P., Fonkalsrud, J., & Crowley, K. (2005). *Structured photographic expressive language test–preschool* (2nd ed.). Janelle Publications.

DeGangi, G. A., Poisson, S., Sickel, R. Z., & Wiener, A. S. (1995). *Infant/toddler symptom checklist: A screening tool for parents*. Therapy Skills Builders.

Dichtelmiller, M. L., Jablon, J. R., Marsden, D. B., & Meisels, S. J. (2014). *The work sampling system* (5th ed.) for Head Start. Pearson Education.

Dodd, B., Hua, Z., Crosbie, S., Holm, A., & Ozanne, A. (2006). *Diagnostic evaluation of articulation and phonology (DEAP)*. Psychological Corporation.

Dunn, D. M. (2018). *Peabody picture vocabulary test* (5th ed.). NCSPearson.

Dunn, W. (2002). *The infant/toddler sensory profile manual*. Psychological Corporation.

Dunn, W. (2014). *Sensory profile 2: User's manual*. Pearson.

Dykes, M. K., & Mruzek, D. W. (2012). *Developmental assessment for the severely handicapped (DASH-3)* (3rd ed.). PRO-ED.

Edwards, S., Letts, C., & Sinka, I. (2011). *The new Reynell developmental language scales*. GL-Assessment.

Ehrler, D. J., & McGhee, R. L. (2008). *Primary test of nonverbal intelligence*. PRO-ED.

Elliott, C. D. (2007). *Differential ability scales* (2nd ed.). Harcourt Assessment.

Epstein, M. H. (2004). *Behavioral and emotional rating scale* (2nd ed.). PRO-ED.

Euler, B. L. (2007). *Emotional disturbance decision tree professional manual*. Psychological Assessment Resources.

Eyberg, S. M., & Pincus, D. (1999). *Eyberg child behavior inventory (ECBI) & Sutter-Eyberg student behavior inventory-revised (SESBI-R)*. Psychological Assessment Resources.

Fantuzzo, J. W., Sutton-Smith, B., Coolahan, K. C., Manz, P., Canning, S., & Debnam, D. (1995). Assessment of play interaction behaviors in young low-income children: Penn Interactive Peer Play Scale. *Early Childhood Research Quarterly, 10*(1), 105–120.

Fenson, L., Marchman, V. A., Thal, D. J., Dale, P. S., Reznick, J. S., & Bates, E. (2007). *MacArthur–Bates communicative development inventories*. Brookes.

Fewell, R. R., & Langley, M. B. (1984). *Developmental activities screening inventory II*. PRO-ED.

Finello, K. M., & Poulsen, M. K. (2018). *Behavioral Assessment of Baby's Emotional & Social Style (BABES) toolkit: Intervention strategies for developmental guidance & support*. WestEd.

Fluharty, N. (2000). *Fluharty preschool speech and language screening test–Second edition (Fluharty-2)*. PRO-ED.

Folio, M. K., & Fewell, R. (2023). *Peabody developmental motor scales: Examiner's manual* (3rd ed.). PRO-ED.

Foster, R., Giddan, J. J., & Stark, J. (1983). *Assessment of children's language comprehension (1983 rev.)*. Riverside Assessments, LLC.

Frankenburg, W. K., Dodds, J., Archer, P., Shapiro, H., & Bresnick, B. (1992). The Denver II: A major revision and restandardization of the Denver Developmental Screening Test. *Pediatrics, 89*(1), 91–97.

Fudala, J. B., & Stegall, S. (2017). *Arizona-4: Arizona articulation and phonology scale, fourth revision*. Western Psychological Services.

Gadow, K., & Sprafkin, J. (2008). *ADHD symptom checklist—4 (ADHD-4)*. Checkmate Plus.

Gadow, K., & Sprafkin, J. (2013). *Child and adolescent symptom inventory-5 (CASI-5)*. Checkmate Plus.

Geffner, D., & Goldman, R. (2010). *Auditory skills assessment*. Pearson Education.

Gesell Institute of Child Development. (2012). *Gesell developmental observation – Revised and Gesell early screener technical report*. Author.

Gilliam, J. E. (2014). *Gilliam autism rating scale* (3rd ed.). PRO-ED.

Gilliam, J. E. (2015). *Attention-deficit/hyperactivity disorder test* ((2nd ed.) ed. [Assessment Instrument].). PRO-ED.

Gilliam, J. E. (2001). *Gilliam Asperger's disorder scale: GADS*. PRO-ED.

Ginsburg, H. P., & Baroody, A. J. (2003). *The test of early mathematics ability* (3rd ed.). PRO-ED.

Gioia, G. A., Isquith, P. K., Guy, S. C., & Kenworthy, L. (2015). *Behavior rating inventory of executive function–Second edition (BRIEF2)*. Psychological Assessment Resources.

Glascoe, F. P., Woods, S. K., & Mills, T. D. (2023). *Parents' evaluation of developmental status, revised*. PEDStest.com, LLC.

Goldman, R., & Fristoe, M. (2015). *Goldman-Fristoe test of articulation 3*. Pearson Education.

Goldstein, S., & Naglieri, J. A. (2009). *ASRS: Autism spectrum rating scales*. Multi-Health Systems.

Goodman, R. (1997). The Strengths and Difficulties Questionnaire: A research note. *Journal of Child Psychology and Psychiatry, 38*(5), 581–586.

Gray, K., Tonge, B. J., Einfeld, S., Gruber, C., & Klein, A. (2018). *DBC2: Developmental behaviour checklist 2 (DBC2) manual*. Western Psychological Services.

Greenspan, S. (2004). *Greenspan social-emotional growth chart [Database record]*. APA PsycTests. https://doi.org/10.1037/t15099-000

Greenspan, S. I., DeGangi, G., & Wieder, S. (2001). *The functional emotional assessment scale (FEAS): For infancy & early childhood*. Interdisciplinary Council on Development & Learning Disorders.

Gresham, F. M., & Elliott, S. N. (1990). *The social skills rating system*. American Guidance Service.

Gresham, F. M., & Elliott, S. N. (2008). *Social skills improvement system (SSIS) rating scales*. Pearson Assessments.

Haley, S. M., Coster, W. J., Dumas, H. M., Fragala-Pinkham, M. A., & Moed, R. (2020). *Pediatric evaluation of disability inventory computer adaptive test (PEDI-CAT)*. Pearson.

Haley, S. M., Coster, W. J., Ludlow, L. H., Haltiwanger, J. T., & Andrellos, P. J. (1992). *Pediatric evaluation of disability inventory (PEDI): Development, standardization and administration manual*. PEDI Research Group, New England Medical Center Hospitals.

Hamaguchi, P., & Ross-Swain, D. (2015). *Receptive, expressive & social communication assessment–elementary*. Western Psychological Services.

Hammill, D. D., Pearson, N. A., & Voress, J. K. (2013). *Developmental test of visual perception* (3rd ed.). PRO-ED.

Hammill, D., & Bryant, B. (2005). *Detroit test of learning aptitude-primary* (3rd ed.). PRO-ED.

Harrison, P. L., & Oakland, T. (2015). *Adaptive behavior assessment system* (3rd ed.). Western Psychological Services.

Hedrick, D. L., Prather, E. M., Tobin, A. R., Allen, D. V., Bliss, L. S., & Rosenberg, L. R. (1984). *Sequenced inventory of communication development–Revised (SICD-R)*. Western Psychological Services.

Henderson, S. E., & Barnett, A. L. (2023). *Movement assessment battery for children* (3rd ed.). NCS Pearson.

Hiskey, M. S. (1966). *Hiskey-Nebraska test of learning aptitude*. Onion College Press.

Hodson, B. (2004). *Hodson assessment of phonological patterns* (3rd ed.). PRO-ED.

Howes, C., & Matheson, C. C. (1992). Sequences in the development of competent play with peers: Social and social pretend play. *Developmental Psychology, 28*, 961–974. https://doi.org/10.1037/0012-1649.28.5.961

Hresko, W. P., Reid, D. K., & Hammill, D. D. (2018). *Test of early language development* (4th ed.). PRO-ED.

Huer, M. B., & Miller, L. (2011). *Examiner's manual of the test of early communication and emerging language (TECEL)*. PRO-ED.

Ilg, F. L., Ames, L. B., Haines, J., & Gillespie, C. (1978). *School readiness: Behavior tests used at the Gesell Institute*. Harper & Row.

Ireton, H. (1992). *Child development inventory*. Behavior Science Systems, Inc.

Ireton, H. (1994). *Infant development inventory*. Behavior Science Systems Inc.

Jelm, J. M. (1990). *Oral-motor feeding rating scale* (1st ed.). Therapy Skill Builders.

Jensen, S. L. (2012). *Early functional communication profile*. Pro-Ed.

Kaufman, A. S., & Kaufman, N. L. (2022). *Kaufman brief intelligence test–Second edition-Revised (KBIT-2-R)*. NCS Pearson.

Kaufman, A. S., & Kaufman, N. L. (1993). *Kaufman survey of early academic and language skills: K-SEALS*. American Guidance Service.

Kaufman, A. S., & Kaufman, N. L. (2018). *Kaufman assessment battery for children-Second edition normative update*. NCS Pearson.

Kaufman, N. (2016). *Kaufman speech praxis test for children*. Pro-Ed.

Khan, L. M., & Lewis, N. P. (2015). *Khan-Lewis phonological analysis, Third edition*. Pearson Education.

Kleiman, L. I. (2003). *Functional communication profile – revised*. LinguiSystems.

Korkman, M., Kirk, U., & Kemp, S. (2007). *NEPSY–Second edition (NEPSY-II)*. Harcourt Assessment.

Krug, D. A., Arick, J. R., & Almond, P. J. (2008). *ASIEP-3: Autism screening instrument for educational planning, 3rd ed*. PRO-ED Inc.

Lachar, D., & Gruber, C. P. (2002). *Personality inventory for children-Second edition*. Multi-Health Systems.

LaFreniere, P. J., & Dumas, J. E. (1995). *Social competence and behavior evaluation: Preschool edition (SCBE)*. Western Psychological Services.

Lambert, N., & Windmiller, M. (1981). *AAMD adaptive behavior scale, school edition*. Test Publisher service.

Langley, M. B., Fewell, R., & Maddox, T. (2010). *Cognitive assessment of young children (CAYC)*. Pro-Ed.

LeBuffe, P. A., & Naglieri, J. A. (2012). *Devereux early childhood assessments for preschool, Second edition (Technical manual)*. Kaplan Early Learning Company.

LeBuffe, P., & Naglieri, J. (2002). *Devereux early childhood assessment–Clinical (DECA-C)*. APA PsycTests. https://doi.org/10.1037/t15185-000

Lee, L. (1971). *Northwestern syntax screening test*. Northwestern University Press.

Lindamood, P. C., & Lindamood, P. (2004). *Lindamood auditory conceptualization test, Third edition*. Pro-Ed.

Linder, T. W. (2008). *Transdisciplinary play-based assessment* (2nd ed.). Paul H. Brookes.

Lippke, B., Dickey, S., Selmar, J., & Soder, A. (1997). *Photo articulation test, Third edition*. Pro-Ed.

Lord, C., Rutter, M., Di Lavore, P., Risi, S., Gotham, K., & Bishop, S. (2012). *Autism diagnostic observation schedule, Second edition (ADOS-2) manual (part I): Modules 1–4*. Western Psychological Services.

Lowe, M., & Costello, A. (1988). *Symbolic play test, Second edition*. GL Assessment.

MacKrain, M., & LeBuffe, P. (2007). *Devereux early childhood assessment for infants and toddlers (DECA-I/T)*. APA PsycTests. https://doi.org/10.1037/t15185-000

Marcott, A. (2009). *Evaluating acquired skills in communication, Third edition*. Pro-Ed.

Mardell, C., & Goldenberg, D. S. (2011). *Speed developmental indicators for the assessment of learning—Fourth edition (Speed DIAL-4)*. Pearson.

Martin, N. A. (2010). *Test of visual-motor skills, Third edition (TVMS-3)*. Western Psychological Services.

Martin, N. A. (2017). *Test of visual perceptual skills* (4th ed.). Academic Therapy Publications.

Martin, N. A., & Brownell, R. (2011b). *Receptive one-word picture vocabulary test-Fourth Edition*. Pro-Ed.

Martin, N. A., & Brownell, R. (2011a). *Expressive one-word picture vocabulary test, Fourth edition*. Pro-Ed.

Martin, N., Brownell, R., & Hamaguchi, P. (2018). *TAPS-4: A language processing skills assessment*. Academic Therapy Publications.

Martin, R. (1988). *The temperament assessment battery for children*. Clinical Psychology Publishing Company.

McCarney, S. B., & House, N. H. (2019). *Attention deficit disorders evaluation dcale–Fifth edition (ADDED-5)*. Hawthorne.

McCarthy, D. (1972). *Manual for the McCarthy scales of children's abilities*. The Psychological Corporation.

McConaughy, S. H., & Achenbach, T. M. (2004). *Manual for the test observation form for ages 2–18*. University of Vermont, Research Center for Children, Youth, & Families.

McGhee, R. L., Di Simoni, F., & Ehrler, D. J. (2007). *TTFC-2: The token test for children*. Pro-Ed.

Meadow, K. P., Getson, P., Lee, C. K., Stamper, L., Karchmer, M. A., Peterson, L. M., & Rudner, L. (1983). *Meadow-Kendall social-emotional assessment inventories for deaf and hearing-impaired students: The revised SEAI manual*. Center for Studies in Education and Human Development.

Meisels, S. J., Dombro, A. L., Marsden, D. B., Weston, D. R., & Jewkes, A. M. (2003). *The ounce scale*. Pearson Early Learning.

Meisels, S. J., Marsden, D. B., Henderson, L. W., & Wiske, M. S. (2019). *The early screening inventory, Third edition*. Pearson Education.

Merrell, K. W. (2002). *Preschool and kindergarten behavior scales-Second edition*. Pro-Ed.

Merrell, K. W. (2011). *Social and emotional assets and resilience scales (SEARS)*. Psychological Assessment Resources.

Miller, J. F., & Paul, R. (1995). *The clinical assessment of language comprehension*. Paul H. Brookes.

Miller, L. J. (1982). *Miller assessment for preschoolers (MAP)*. Foundation for Knowledge in Development.

Miller, L. J. (1993). *FirstSTEp: Screening test for evaluating preschoolers (FirstSTEp)*. APA PsycTests. https://doi.org/10.1037/t15088-000

Miller, L. J. (2006). *Miller function and participation scales: Examiner's manual*. Psychological Corporation.

Miller, L., Gillam, R. B., & Peña, E. (2001). *Dynamic assessment and intervention: Improving children's narrative abilities*. Paul H. Brookes.

Monteiro, M. J., & Stegall, S. (2018). *Monteiro interview guidelines for diagnosing the autism spectrum, Second edition (MIGDAS-2)* (2nd ed., Vol. 2). WPS Publishing.

Mullen, E. M. (1995). *Mullen scales of early learning*. American Guidance Service.

Myles, B. S., Simpson, R. L., & Bock, S. J. (2001). *Asperger syndrome diagnostic scale*. Pro-ed.

Hardin, B. J., Peisner-Feinberg, E. S., & Weeks, S. W. (2005). *The learning accomplishment profile-diagnostic (LAP-D)* (3rd ed.). Kaplan Early Learning Company.

Newborg, J. (2020). *Battelle developmental inventory, Third edition: Examiner's manual*. Riverside Assessments, LLC.

Nihira, K., Foster, R., Shellhaas, M., & Leland, H. (1993). *AAMD adaptive behavior scale: Revised edition*. American Association on Mental Deficiency.

Nurss, J. R., & McGauvran, M. E. (1995). *Metropolitan readiness test, Sixth edition (MRT6)*. Pearson.

Olswang, L., Stoel-Gammon, C., Coggins, T., & Carpenter, R. (1987). *Assessing prelinguistic and early linguistic behaviors in developmentally young children*. University of Washington Press.

Parham, L. D., Ecker, C. L., Kuhaneck, H., Henry, D. A., & Glennon, T. J. (2021). *Sensory processing measure* (Second ed.). Western Psychological Service.

Pearson, N. A., Patton, J. R., & Mruzek, D. M. (2016). *Adaptive behavior diagnostic scale*. Riverside.

Provence, S., & Apfel, N. (2001). *Infant-Toddler and family instrument*. Paul H. Brookes Publishing Co., Inc.

Provence, S., Erickson, J., Vater, S., Palmeri, S., Pruett, K., & Rosinia, J. (2016). *Infant-Toddler developmental assessment, Second edition: Administration manual*. Pro-ed.

Reid, D. K., Hresko, W. P., & Hammill, D. D. (2018). *Test of early reading ability—Fourth edition (TERA-4)*. Pro-ed.

Reid, D. K., Hresko, W. P., Hammill, D. D., & Wiltshire, S. (1991). *Test of early reading ability: Deaf or hard of hearing*. Pro-ed.

Reuter, J., Katoff, L., & Gruber, C. (2000). *Kent inventory of developmental skills (KIDS)*. Western Psychological Services.

Reynell, J. (1979). *Manual for the Reynell-Zinkin scales, developmental scales for young visually handicapped children, Part 1 mental development*. NFER-Nelson Publishing Company.

Reynolds, C. R., & Kamphaus, R. W. (2015a). *BASC-3 behavioral and emotional screening system manual*. Pearson.

Reynolds, C. R., & Kamphaus, R. W. (2015c). *Reynolds intellectual assessment scales, Second edition*. Psychological Assessment Resources.

Reynolds, C. R. (2007). *Koppitz developmental scoring system for the bender gestalt test (KOPPITZ-2)*. Pro-ed.

Reynolds, C. R., & Kamphaus, R. W. (2007). *TIWRE: Test of irregular word reading efficiency.* Psychological Assessment Resources.

Reynolds, C. R., & Kamphaus, R. W. (2015b). *Behavior assessment system for children* (3rd ed.). NCS Pearson, Inc. (BASC–3)

Richman, N. (1988). *Preschool behavior checklist.* Academic Therapy Publications.

Riley, G. D. (2009). *Stuttering severity instrument* (4th ed.). PRO-ED.

Robins, D. L., Fein, D., & Barton, M. (2009). *Modified checklist for autism in toddlers, revised, with follow-up (M-CHAT-R/F).* Lineage.

Roid, G. H. (2003). *Stanford-Binet intelligence scales–Fifth edition.* Riverside Publishing.

Roid, G. H., & Sampers, J. L. (2004). *Merrill-Palmer-Revised scales of development (MPR) [Database record].* APA PsycTests. https://doi.org/10.1037/t06030-000

Roid, G. H., Miller, L. J., Pomplun, M., & Koch, C. (2013). *Leiter international performance scale-Third edition.* Stoelting Company.

Rossetti, L. (2006). *The Rossetti Infant-Toddler language scale.* Linguisystems.

Rutter, M., Bailey, A., & Lord, C. (2003). *The social communication questionnaire: Manual.* Western Psychological Services.

Rutter, M., Le Couteur, A., & Lord, C. (2003). *Autism diagnostic interview-revised.* Western Psychological Services.

Schafer, S. D., & Moersch, M. S. (1981). *Developmental programming for infants and young children, Revised edition.* University of Michigan Press ELT. https://doi.org/10.3998/mpub.8136

Schopler, E., Lansing, M. D., Reichler, R. J., & Marcus, L. M. (2005). *Psychoeducational profile: PEP-3: TEACCH individualized psychoeducational assessment for children with autism spectrum disorders.* Pro-ed.

Schopler, E., Reichler, R. J., & Renner, B. R. (2010). *The childhood autism rating scale (CARS).* Western Psychological Services.

Schrank, F. A., McGrew, K., & Mather, N. (2015). *Woodcock-Johnson IV tests of early cognitive and academic development.* Riverside.

Secord, W. A., & Donohue, J. S. (2013). *Clinical assessment of articulation and phonology – Second edition (CAAP-2).* WPS.

Seymour, H. N., Roeper, T., & de Villiers, J. G. (2018). *Diagnostic evaluation of language variation-norm referenced (DELV-NR).* The Psychological Corporation. [Republished 2018, Sun Prairie, WI: Ventris Learning.]

Sherman, E. M. S., & Brooks, B. L. (2015). *Child and adolescent memory profile.* Psychological Assessment Resources.

Siegel, B. (2004). *Pervasive developmental disorders screening test, second edition (PDDST-II).* NCS Pearson.

Simeonsson, R. J., Huntington, G. S., Short, R. J., & Ware, W. B. (1982). The Carolina Record of Individual Behavior: Characteristics of Handicapped Infants and Children. *Topics in Early Childhood Special Education, 2*(2), 43–55. https://doi.org/10.1177/027112148200200209

Slosson, R. L. (2017). *Slosson intelligence test-Fourth edition (SIT-4).* Slosson Educational Publication. http://www.slosson.com/onlinecatalogstore_c394797.html

Smith, A. J., & Johnson, R. E. (1977). *Smith-Johnson nonverbal performance scale.* Western Psychological Services.

Sparrow, S. S., Balla, D. A., & Cicchetti, D. V. (1998). *Vineland social-emotional early childhood scales.* American Guidance Service.

Sparrow, S. S., Cicchetti, D. V., & Saulnier, C. A. (2016). *Vineland-3: Vineland adaptive behavior scales.* PsychCorp.

Squires, J., Bricker, D., & Twombly, E. (2015). *Ages & stages questionnaires®: Social-emotional, Second edition (ASQ®): A Parent-Completed Child Monitoring System for Social-Emotional Behaviors*. Paul H. Brookes Publishing Co.

Squires, J., & Bricker, D. (2009). *Ages & stages questionnaires, Third edition (ASQ-3): A parent-completed child monitoring system*. Paul H. Brookes Publishing Co.

Stillman, R. D. (1984). *The Callier-Azusa scale*. Callier Center for Communication Disorders.

Stone, W. L., Coonrod, E. E., Pozdol, S. L., & Turner, L. M. (2003). The parent interview for autism-clinical version (PIA-CV): A measure of behavioral change for young children with autism. *Autism: The International Journal of Research and Practice, 7*(1), 9–30. https://doi.org/10.1177/1362361303007001003

Stone, W., & Ousley, O. Y. (2008). *Screening tool for autism in toddlers and young children (STAT)*. Vanderbilt University.

Stroud, L., Foxcroft, C., Green, E., Bloomfield, S., Cronje, J., Hurter, K., . . . Venter, D. (2016). *Griffiths scales of child development 3rd ed. Part I: Overview, development and psychometric properties*. Hogrefe.

Stuberg, W. A., Dehne, P. R., Miedaner, J. A., & White, P. (1992). *Milani-Comparetti motor development screening test*. Munroe-Meyer Institute for Genetics & Rehabilitation.

Sundberg, M. L. (2016). *VB-MAPP: Verbal behavior milestones assessment and placement program: A language and social skills assessment program for children with autism or other developmental disabilities (Guide) 2nd Edition*. AVB Press.

Torgesen, J. K., & Bryant, B. R. (2004). *Test of phonological awareness—Second edition: Plus*. Pro-Ed.

Ulrich, D. A. (2019). *The test of gross motor development–3rd edition (TGMD-3)*. Pro-Ed.

University of Oregon. (2023). *8th edition of the dynamic indicators of basic early literacy education (DIBELS): Administration and scoring guide, 2023 edition*. Author. https://dibels.uoregon.edu

Uzgiris, I. C., & Hunt, J. M. (1975). *Ordinal scales of psychological development—1975*. University of Illinois Press.

Voress, J. K., Maddox, T., & Hammill, D. D. (2012). *Developmental assessment of young children* (2nd ed.). Pro-Ed.

VORT Corporation. (2010). *Hawaii early learning profile: 3-6 years* (2nd ed.). VORT Corporation.

Wagner, R. K., Torgesen, J. K., Rashotte, C. A., & Pearson, N. A. (2013). *Comprehensive test of phonological processing* (2nd ed.). Pro-Ed.

Walker, H. M., Severson, H. H., & Feil, E. G. (1995). *Early screening project: A proven child-find process*. Sopris West.

Wallace, G., & Hammill, D. D. (2013). *Comprehensive receptive and expressive vocabulary test—Third edition (CREVT-3)*. Pro-Ed.

Webster, R. E. (2009). *Test of information processing skills*. ATP Assessments.

Wechsler, D. (2012). *Wechsler preschool and primary scale of intelligence—Fourth edition*. The Psychological Corporation.

Westby, C. E. (2000). A scale for assessing development of children's play. In K. Giltin-Weiner, A. Sandgrund, & C. Schaefer (Eds.), *Play diagnosis and assessment* (pp. 15–57). Wiley.

Wetherby, A. M., & Prizant, B. M. (2002). *Communication and symbolic behavior scales developmental profile, first normed edition (CSBS DP)*. APA PsycTests.

Wiig, E. H., Secord, W. A., & Semel, E. (2020). *Clinical evaluation of language fundamentals preschool–3*. Pearson Education.

Williams, K. T. (2019). *Expressive vocabulary test* (3rd ed.) [Measurement instrument]). NCS Pearson.

Wong, V., Hui, L.-H. S., Lee, W.-C., Leung, L.-S. J., Ho, P.-K. P., Lau, W.-L. C., Fung, C.-W., & Chung, B. (2004). A modified screening tool for autism (Checklist for Autism in Toddlers [CHAT-23]) for Chinese children. *Pediatrics, 114,* e166–e176.

Woodcock, R. W., McGrew, K. S., & Mather, N. (2014). *Woodcock-Johnson IV tests of achievement.* Riverside.

Zeitlin, S. (1985). *Coping inventory: A measure of adaptive behavior.* Scholastic Testing Service.

Zeitlin, S., Szczepanski, M., & Williamson, G. G. (1988). *Early coping inventory.* Scholastic Testing Service.

Zimmerman, I. L., Steiner, V. G., & Pond, R. E. (2011). *Preschool language scales—Fifth edition (PLS-5).* Pearson. https://doi.org/10.1037/t15141-000

Index

Printed and bound by CPI Group (UK) Ltd, Croydon, CR0 4YY

07/07/2026

14916212-0003